HEALTHY TEX-MEX

The South Texas Slim Down

Copyright © 2013 Juan C. Prieto M.D.
All rights reserved.

ISBN 10: 1492933295
ISBN 13: 9781492933298

HEALTHY TEX-MEX

The South Texas Slim Down

*Juan C. Prieto M.D. • Text by Shelby Killion R.D. •
Authored with Kimberly J. Norman*

TABLE OF CONTENTS

INTRODUCTION 1

Chapter 1	HOW TO USE THIS BOOK 3
	• GEMS- Goals Equal My Success 4
	• Slim GEMS 8

Chapter 2	Fuel Up With Premium Grade 9
	• Carbohydrates 9
	• Fiber 10
	• Fruits and Vegetables 10
	• Protein 11
	• Fat 11
	• Vitamins and Minerals 13
	• Water 13
	• Slim GEMS 14

Chapter 3	Calories! 15
	• Secrets of Weight Loss 17
	• Time for goal setting! 18
	• Slim GEMS 21

TABLE OF CONTENTS

Chapter 4 — What Do I See? 23
- Slim GEMS 24

Chapter 5 — Mastering Grocery Shopping and Portion Control 25
- Reading labels 26
- Slim GEMS 28

Chapter 6 — Emotional Eating 29
- Celebrate! 29
- Lonely, Sad or Mad 31
- Journal Entry 31
- Finish Your Plate! 31
- Stressed! 32
- Cravings! 32
- My Food Journal Before 34
- My Food Journal After 36
- Slim GEMS 37

Chapter 7 — What is for Dinner? 39
- Life Before the South Texas Slim Down 40
- Life After the South Texas Slim Down 40
- An example of enjoying healthy meals with a busy week: 42
- Slim GEMS 44

Chapter 8 — Recipes 45
- How to use the recipe section of the book 45
- Sides 47
- Eggs 66
- Poultry 69
- Beef 76

TABLE OF CONTENTS

- Fish · 82
- Pork · 84
- Vegetarian · 85

Chapter 9   LET'S BURN THOSE TORTILLAS! · 89
- How to use the fitness section of the book · 89
- Workout Instructions: · 90
- Week 1 · 91
- Week 2 · 97
- Week 3 · 103
- Week 4 · 109

Appendix · 115
- A: Keeping Track Keeps me On Track (Food Diary, Physical Activity, GEMS for the Week, Menu Planning) · 115
- B: BMI Chart · 119
- C: Websites, Apps and Other Great Resources · 120
- Websites · 120
- Apps · 120
- D: How to Read Nutritional Label · 121
- Healthy Pre-packed Snack Ideas · 122

Endnotes · 125

HEATHLY TEX-MEX: THE SOUTH TEXAS SLIM DOWN TEAM

MEDICAL EDITOR IN CHIEF
JUAN C PRIETO, M.D.

NURTITION EDITOR
SHELBY KILLION, R.D.

EDITOR-IN-CHIEF, SENIOR EDITOR
KIMBERLY NORMAN

CHEF
MARIO MANTILLA

FITNESS CONTRIBUTOR
LAUREN FLORES

PHOTOGRAPHER
ASHLEY JONES

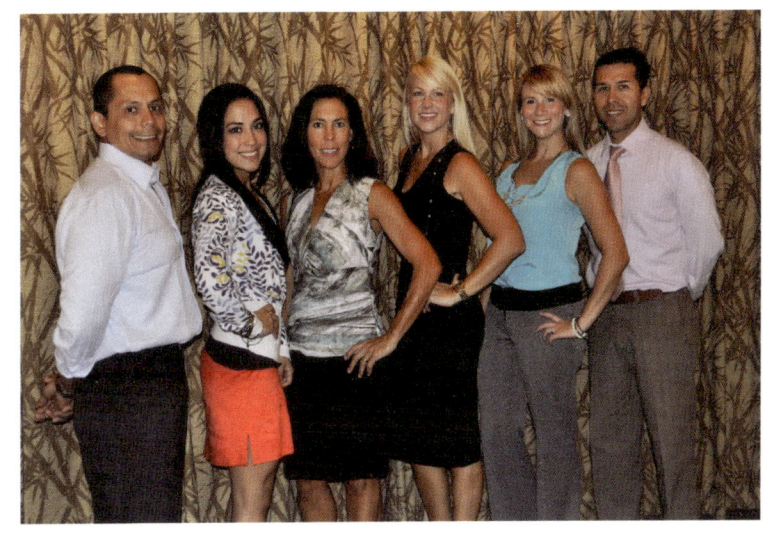

INTRODUCTION

Juan C. Prieto, M.D.

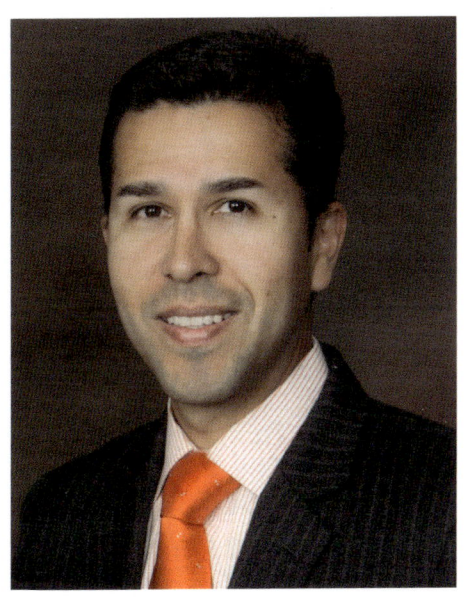

Dr. Juan Prieto is a physician specialized in pediatric urology who was trained at Miami Children's Hospital/University of Miami and Children's Medical Center of Dallas/University of Texas Southwestern Medical Center. Since 2009, Dr. Prieto has practiced pediatric urology in South Texas (McAllen, Corpus Christi, and San Antonio). Furthermore, he has served as an Expert Peer Reviewer for the Journal of Urology, Journal of Pediatric Urology, International Brazilian Journal of Urology, and Frontiers in Pediatric Urology. Dr. Prieto is a member of the American Urological Association and the Society for Pediatric Urology.

Why We Wrote This Book

In my clinics, I come across patients and their families who have tried diets in the past to attempt to lose weight, but the weight never stays off. Similarly, I met many people that recognize their overweight problem but have no guidance how to grocery shop, eat or cook in a healthier manner. This epidemic in South Texas (and throughout our country) reveals an unfulfilled need- South Texans need a diet book that considers their culture, their food, and their lifestyle. We have met this need in our book.

Our focus is on one's overall health, but we approach it in a very personable way. You can find other diet books that will have "healthier" recipes that may help you lose weight faster, but we are offering a diet book that is full of "baby-steps" that will not intimidate anyone. You will experience success and have fun doing it! More than that, you will find the recipes so enjoyable that they will make their way into your weekly meal planning. Furthermore, we are offering you tips on how to grocery shop and how to exercise at home in a progressive manner.

So, turn the page and begin your new adventure into a healthier lifestyle and a happier life. Start losing weight eating what you like…Tex-Mex and South Texas cuisine.

CHAPTER 1: HOW TO USE THIS BOOK

Shelby Killion, R.D.

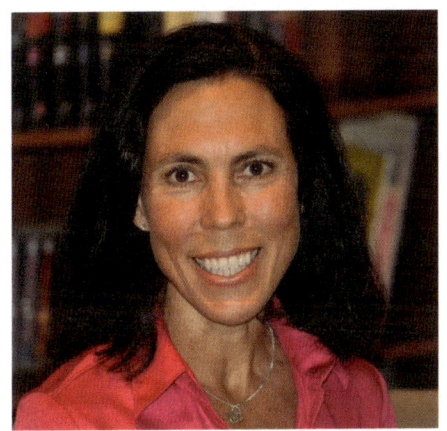

Shelby Killion is a registered and licensed dietitian since 1988 with a passion for helping people achieve their goals of a healthier lifestyle with weight management, prevention and management of chronic disease. She is the owner of Food & Fit Solutions, president of the Corpus Christi Academy of Nutrition and Dietetics and volunteers with local organizations to promote good health. She loves practicing what she preaches by making good healthy food choices and staying physically active.

> Bel,
> I love that you always strive to be the best you can be.
> God bless
> Shelby

Gem – something that is valued for its perfection.

GEMS- Goals Equal My Success

As a South Texan, you enjoy a culture rich in family tradition, celebration and flavorful food. Although perhaps hard to envision, a healthier lifestyle does not require sacrificing all the things that are important to you. Keeping family tradition, celebrating life and eating healthier flavorful food in smaller portions while establishing exercise routines will lead to weight loss and a number of health benefits including decreased risks of diabetes, heart disease, stroke and even some cancers.[1] On a more daily basis, you will experience higher-quality sleep, increased energy, reduced indigestion and I dare say, regular bowel movements.[2-5] And you can enjoy these benefits even before attaining your ideal weight.[6] After such improvements, it will be hard to imagine living any other way.

Take this challenge one step at a time. Although seemingly insignificant, small changes are essential because they lead to long-term habits. Give yourself time with a new routine and in a month or two, it will become your new norm.[7] Think back to a diet you have tried in the past. Did you start full throttle and then by day three, toss it out? Usually, reason being the **fad diet was too restrictive**. By focusing on a few manageable goals at a time, you will find that change is possible and before you know it, you won't even miss that nighttime bowl of ice cream.

Before going any further, I want you to stop and think about something very important. You want to lose weight. And if the figures are right, you're part of the 54 percent of people who do.[8] Remember that the safest way to lose weight is gradually – roughly 1-2 pounds per week. Rapid weight loss may seem ideal but in most of these cases, people regain the weight they lost, plus more. This fact should be proof enough that the quickest method is not necessarily the best one.

It is easy to understand the need for a map when you are traveling or on a journey. This same idea applies when starting your health journey. Spend time writing out your goals-they will be your roadmap to success.

> If you don't know where you are going, you'll end up someplace else.
>
> Yogi Berra

First, think of your **long term goals**. What realistic results do you want in three months, six months. Second, find an **accountability partner**. This person may be your spouse, a family member, a friend or a even a registered dietitian. Someone you can talk to and will give you the support and accountability you need. Third, plan for **non-food rewards** at certain points of your journey. After one month of hard work, treat yourself to something nice: a new book, a manicure, or maybe a new fishing rod. The point is to celebrate your success!

HOW TO USE THIS BOOK

Maybe you are thinking something along these lines:

Long Term Goal In 3 Months	Long Term Goal In 6 Months	My Accountability Partner	My Celebration Will Be
By March 31st I will be 20 pounds lighter.	By June 30th I will be 40 pounds lighter.	My sister will help me when I need extra motivation, help me when I get off track and celebrate my success with me.	I will fit into my old jeans and go dancing.

You know now where you want to be and when, now think about **how** you are going to get there. Getting there takes action. These action steps will be your **GEMS**. Think about it this way **Goals Equal My Success** and your precious GEMS will get you where you want to be.

You, of course, can add personalized goals in areas you know need attention as well. Work on three GEMS at a time. Your Keeping Track Keeps Me on Track form (Appendix A) includes a place to write your GEMS for each week.

> At the end of each section of the book, you will be given your Slim GEMS. These are action steps that are basic to your success in establishing a healthy lifestyle and losing the weight.

Here is an example to help your thinking process.

Specific and Realistic Action	Plan for Obstacles	Accomplished? What Now?
I will be eat at home for breakfast & dinner and pack my lunch for work with eating only one restaurant meal.	I will shop for easy meal options and pack the night before. I will preportion food for the freezer that I can grab when short on time. When asked by coworkers, I will say I can join them on Friday.	Yes accomplished 5 days of the week. The weekend, ate out for two meals. Next time will not eat out during week and allow two reastaurant meals on weekend choosing lean options.
I will drink 8 cups of water a day and cut back on soda to one every other day.	I will buy water bottles and keep cold. I will get rid of my sodas from the house. If my craving is super strong, after 10 minute wait, I will allow a couple of sips if craving still.	I got up to 6 cups every day and 8 cups on one day. I was able to decrease my sodas to only two a week. Now I am ready for 8 cups of water and no sodas.
I will walk for 20 minutes 4/week.	On busy days, I will split it up to two 10 minute walks. If bad weather, I will walk on my treadmill.	Yes accomplished. Now I am ready to walk at a faster pace and will continue 4/week for another week.

You will need quick and easy access to your GEMS, so be sure to make multiple copies. Increase your chances for success by reading your goals every morning and evening.[9] Simply writing them out once and putting them out of sight, will not lead to results. An important question to ask yourself throughout the day is: Does this take me closer to my goal? You will find if you honestly ask this question, the donut that you are about to grab from the break room does not seem as appealing anymore. Knowing that the donut does not get you closer to your goal and after thinking about it, you realize you are not even hungry. You feel confident about your decision to walk right past the donut.

> We are what we repeatedly do. Excellence, then, is not an act but a habit.
>
> — Aristotle

Believe in yourself that you can accomplish your goals. **Visualizing taking positive steps towards your goal will help you actually attain that goal**. Studies have shown that those who visualized their positive action steps had better chances of reaching their end result than those that visualized the end result.[10] Practically speaking, this means seeing yourself walking past the dessert area without reaching for one or visualizing writing a list for the grocery store and not walking down the chip isle because chips are not on the list.

These practices may seem strange at first, simply because they are out of your routine. However, your subconscious mind is a powerful thing, so use it to help and not to hinder you. Read your action steps and visualize yourself doing them, always considering whether your actions are conducive to reaching your goal. Remember that within your action steps you also have some flexibility, so you don't always have to pass up the dessert section of your favorite restaurant.

Chapter 1: SLIM GEMS

- ◆ I will continue reading how lifestyle changes including healthy food choices, portion control and physical activity leads to weight management, decrease chances for certain diseases as well as improve quality of life.
- ◆ I will focus on how a healthy lifestyle can be gained by one step at a time.
- ◆ Long-term goals for 3 months and 6 months need to be identified and written down as well as identifying an accountability partner and a plan to celebrate success.
- ◆ GEMS – an acronym for **Goals Equal My Success**. These precious GEMS will be your focus in order to achieve the long term results. GEMS are specific, realistic and a thought is given to how to deal with obstacles with an evaluation at the end to see if accomplished and what next.
- ◆ Goals should be visible and read routinely.
- ◆ Visualize yourself following through with the action steps.

CHAPTER 2:
FUEL UP WITH PREMIUM GRADE

If you knew that the premium grade fuel would increase your car's performance, extend its life and require less repair costs, would you use it? If you knew that a healthy lifestyle would improve your health, extend your life and require less healthcare costs, would you do it? I hope you jumped up with your fist in the air as you shouted, yes!

Carbohydrates

A healthy lifestyle includes eating nutrient rich foods (the premium grade fuel) that supply the balance of macronutrients-carbohydrates, protein and fat- with the vitamins and minerals and proper hydration that your body needs.

Wholesome carbohydrates are found in whole grains, legumes like pinto beans, fresh fruit, vegetables, and low-fat dairy. Your body needs them to provide energy, vitamins and minerals, and fiber. The fact is that the average American diet consists of the not-so-healthy carbohydrates from sugar and highly refined grains including soda and sweetened drinks, cake and pastries, chips and fried potatoes.[12] Here are some examples that may help you see the lack of nutrition in these choices: Wheat comes from the field with its bran, germ and endosperm intact which supply the vitamins, minerals and fiber that promote good health. However, when we eat the refined wheat products like white bread or chips, the health benefits from the bran and germ are missing. On the other hand, whole wheat retains all of these nutrient rich parts of the wheat and therefore is better for you. Similarly, a potato comes from the field rich in fiber from the skin and no unhealthy fats. As it is processed into French fried potatoes the fiber is lost and now

> "The first wealth is health."
>
> Emerson

contains a substantial amount of fat and in many cases the unhealthy type of fat. Fresh fruit contain an abundance of good nutrition including fiber, vitamins and minerals and phytonutrients-disease fighting compounds. Yet when we only drink the juice, the fiber is missing. Take it another step further and the juice drink that many people drink is just flavored sugar water that lacks all the amazing qualities of the fresh fruit. The point to take home is **the closer to nature the healthier**!

Fiber

The benefits of including dietary fiber are numerous ranging from helping control blood sugars and blood lipids like cholesterol, to maintaining regular bowel movements and keeping you full longer.[13] Striving for the recommended 25-35 grams of fiber per day can be reached with six servings of wholesome carbohydrates, two to three fruits, and three to four non-starchy vegetables. Increasing the fiber in your diet gradually is crucial to allow for your digestive system to adjust. And a must is to drink enough fluids-water, water, water! The added benefit of keeping you full longer will be a big plus to your weight loss efforts.

Fruits and Vegetables

Fresh fruits and vegetables offer health benefits you do not want to miss. The varying flavors and textures that you will add to your plate will not only supply you with bountiful nutrients that help fight chronic disease but will give your taste buds a welcomed surprise.

Think about the fruits and vegetables you and your family eat. How many are on that list? Are they the same ones over and over? I challenge you to try a new fruit or vegetable this week. Will it be blueberries on your morning cereal or kiwi slices on your salad or red and yellow peppers with your chicken or grape tomatoes as a snack? You begin to eat these foods and find that you don't miss the chips that you replaced. You may even find your child begins to try these foods as well because you are eating them.

Protein

Protein, another macronutrient, is necessary for many functions as well as promoting lean body mass. Daily protein intake supplies your body with the essential amino acids-the building blocks of protein. Studies show, like fiber, it will help keep you full longer in which helps your weight loss efforts.[14] High quality protein is found in lean beef, chicken, turkey, pork, fish, tofu, eggs, and low-fat cheese. The cuts of meat and the preparation method are important points to note.

Beef cuts with 10 grams of total fat per 3 ounce portion are lean like sirloin, top round; 95 percent lean ground beef, flank steak, and tenderloin. Removing the skin of chicken or turkey is ideal. Eggs provide great nutrition and one a day can be included in a healthy diet by the American Heart Association guidelines. Cheese is a major ingredient of most Mexican foods and by choosing wisely can continue to be. A tip is to choose cheeses that have 5-6 grams of fat per ounce like mozzarella, 2% cheddar and 2% Mexican Blend, queso fresco skim, quest Oaxaca and panela skim. A goal is to plan for a lean protein source with every meal and most planned snacks.

Tortilla Trimmer

Lean Beef

-sirloin

top round

-95% lean ground beef

-flank steak

-tenderloin

Fat

Fat is vital for absorption of fat soluble vitamins, protection of cell membranes as well as many other functions. The appealing flavors and textures they offer cannot be denied. Along with protein and fiber, they help keep you full longer as well.[15] The key is to choose unsaturated fats that improve health and to avoid saturated and trans fat that are linked to increased cholesterol and triglycerides, both of which increase your chances for heart disease.[16]

Excellent Choices	Poor Choices
Canola oil	Whole fat dairy
olive oil	butter
nuts	fatty meat
avocados	stick margarine
ground flaxseed	partially hydrogenated oil
	sour cream
	gravy
	fatty starches like biscuits
	flour tortillas

When trying to lose weight portions are important with any fat due to the concentrated calories. A slice of avocado is an excellent choice but eating one half cup of guacamole can add 200 calories to your meal. By *aiming for one fat per meal*, **you can decide between the dressing on the salad or the olive oil in your vegetables**. Your body also needs essential fatty acids called omega-3 fatty acids which can be found in fatty fish like salmon, lake trout, mackerel and halibut. The Dietary Guidelines for Americans, 2010 encourage eight ounces of seafood per week. If you do not care for seafood, talk with your doctor about an omega-3 fatty acid supplement.

The macronutrients, carbohydrates, protein and fats are digested at varying rates. Therefore, combining these nutrients at mealtime and snack time will increase your satiety for longer periods of time. Carbohydrates take about 1-2 hours to digest, protein about 2-3 hours and fats 3-4 hours. Ideally you can plan to *eat every 4-5 hours to fuel your body evenly throughout the day.*

Vitamins and Minerals

Vitamins and minerals are micronutrients protect our long-term health like the potassium in bananas helping control blood pressure[17] and calcium and Vitamin D for bone health[18]. There is not one food that contains everything we need. For example, beef is an excellent source of iron but does not contain Vitamin C and oranges are an excellent source of Vitamin C but do not contain iron. **Balance and variety are essential** to getting the required micronutrients. Knowing that there is a great chance of not consuming all the necessary vitamins and minerals needed on a daily basis, a multi vitamin and mineral is a good insurance plan. When shopping for a supplement, a general rule is to buy one geared for you and with USP (United States Pharmacopeia) on the label that shows the quality, purity and potency of the supplement has been checked.

> **Tortilla Trimmer:**
>
> If you cut out 450 calories a day you could lose 4 pounds in one month and 46 pounds in a year. Passing up the soda might be worth the effort!

Water

As elementary as it seems, remember your body needs water. In fact, your body is about 60% water, which needs to be replaced all the time. The amount of fluid your body needs varies from person to person depending on your activity level, the climate, your sweat rate. But it can be determined by a simple question-what is the color of your urine? Clear? You may be drinking too much. Dark yellow and you may not be drinking enough. Light yellow color and you may be just right! Yes, you can hydrate with other liquids but these often contain calories, additives, and too much caffeine. Americans have been known to consume an average 450 calories from sweetened beverages per day! Is it the cheap fuel or the premium grade you want to feed your body! You are in the drivers seat…start making healthier choices today!

Chapter 2 SLIM GEMS

A combination of carbohydrates, protein and fats are required by your body along with vitamins, minerals and water. Fresh whole foods are the best sources with focusing on balance of lean protein, wholesome whole grains, fresh array of colorful fresh fruit and vegetables and low-fat dairy and keeping in mind the need for moderation.

- I will read reliable information to learn what my body really needs. I will read my goal card with the following information everyday to start believing my food choices affect my health and how I feel.
- I will balance carbohydrates, protein and fats at meal time. One-half of my plate will be vegetables and fruit, the other half will be lean protein and the other whole grain. I will include a healthy fat with my meals.
- I will plan to eat healthy snacks like yogurt without added sugar, fresh fruit with low-fat string cheese, boiled egg and baby carrots when hungry in between meals.
- I will eat every 4-5 hours and include a healthy snack during longer gaps.
- I will increase my fruit serving by one until I eat three a day in place of a processed starch like chips.
- I will increase my vegetables by trying a different colored vegetable at each meal.
- I will switch my sweetened beverage for water at least one time a day until I can avoid all sweetened beverages.
- I will take a multi vitamin and mineral daily and will place it by my toothbrush to remind me.
- I will choose one fat

CHAPTER 3:
CALORIES!

Weight management is all about balance! Imagine a seesaw and one side is calories in and the other side is calories out. Tilt one way by eating more calories than you burn, and you will gain weight. Tilt it the other way by eating fewer calories than you burn, and surprise you will lose weight. I know that is somewhat oversimplified, but sometimes the simpler the better. Striving to consume fewer calories than you burn, but not too little, is your goal.

> The secret about getting ahead is getting started.
>
> Mark Twain

Understand your body requires a certain number of calories to simply live, which is your resting metabolic rate (RMR). The extra movement you demand on the body is your activity factor. So the more active you are, the more calories you require. Also, affecting your calorie requirements are body size, lean body mass, and genetics.

An easy formula to use is to find your **healthy weight** (refer to chart in **Appendix B**) and **multiply that by 10** and that will be your **RMR** and add for your activity level.
Refer to the table below to find your activity level.

Add 20-40% for sedentary
40-60% for moderately active
60-80% high activity level

- If you are a 5'3" woman and work at a desk job 8-5pm
  Healthy Weight is 126 x 10= 1,260 + 30% = 1,680 calories required for weight maintenance

- If you are a 5'6" man and work as a tile setter. Healthy Weight is 158 x 10 = 1,580 + 60% = 2,634 calories required for weight maintenance

> My healthy weight _____ x 10= _____ + (activity level)= your calories required for weight maintenance

To lose one pound of weight you must eat 3,500 calories less than what your body requires over a period of time. **Cutting out 250 calories per day would allow .5 pound of weight loss per week and 26 pounds in one year. Cutting out 500 calories per day would allow 1 pound of weight per week and 52 pounds in one year.** This may not be as quick as you would like or as fast as some of the current diets on the market, but it is something you could do for the long haul and therefore actually reach and maintain your goal.

Now that you have determined your calorie budget, you want to make a plan of spending it wisely with nutrient rich foods that will help keep you full longer and provide long-term health benefits.

> **Tortilla Trimmer:**
> To lose one pound of weight you must eat 3,500 calories less

Not one plan fits everyone. The plan that you are able to stick with for the long run is the plan that will work for you. Don't be discouraged if you have not been successful with certain diets. They might not have been the right fit. If you have fallen for the latest fad, you were at a disadvantage. Because fad diets are so restrictive, they do not set you up for long-term success. Twenty-four plus years of counseling has given me some insight to what works and what does not. Some people ask for the secret of weight loss, so I am going to let you in on the secrets of the trade:

SECRETS OF WEIGHT LOSS

If you are "on a diet" then soon you will be "off the diet."

>Secret: Start living a healthy life by eating nutrient rich foods, and smaller portions and become more active.

I will start tomorrow.

>Starting tomorrow implies it is something so drastic you want to put it off.

I don't know why I can't lose weight, I don't even eat breakfast.

>Secret: Identify an action you can take today and imagine doing it for the long haul.

>Secret: Be mindful of what you are putting in your mouth.
>You may be surprised to find that although you do not sit and eat a breakfast, your morning coffee with sugar and creamer and a sweetbread that you ate midmorning add up to 400 calories.

The scale has not budged even though I am walking 30 minutes every other day.

>Secret: A 30 minute walk may burn an extra 200 calories, which can be consumed in a couple bites of your kid's leftover hamburger and fries.
>**Look at physical activity as what our bodies are meant to be doing, not a ticket to be able to eat more.**

I get a big gulp in the morning, but it lasts me all day long.

> Secret: Liquid calories are sneaky because they do not make you feel full, and you don't make adjustment to your food quantities when consumed. Don't waste your calories on beverages, save it for the foods you love most.

I can't do without a little sweet after meals.

> Secret: Taste buds adjust! Avoiding sweets for a time will allow the taste of sugar to be more intense, and your desire to lessen.

I have to have my………..

> Secret: You may feel afraid of change but take on an achievable goal and set your mind to the positive results you will gain. Before long you are living life and never missing that old habit because your new habit is much more rewarding.

You can follow a calorie controlled diet, my plate guidelines, cutting portions in half, no snacking between meals or the suggestions offered in this book. Whatever plan you follow you must start with goal setting.

Time for goal setting!

Begin by monitoring what types of food you are eating and how much you are eating. Many free apps and websites can provide the help needed to determine how many calories you are consuming. If you like technology, use it to your advantage by recording all foods and beverages consumed. Your eyes will be opened to areas needing improvement due to concentrated calories, excessive fat and seductive sugar. If technology is not your friend, then use a piece of paper to record what you eat! It is important to note **what, how much** and **why** in regards to food and beverages. If you notice, many times you answer the question why with "because she offered", "because it was there"," because that is what I usually do when I watch TV" then you know what areas of your life need attention.

Realize your body needs fuel, and that fuel comes from the calories in our food. Your body runs best if those calories are supplied evenly throughout the day, not sporadically. If you are not eating regularly your body adapts by conserving and storing more, which means no weight loss. Starting the day by breaking your nighttime fast with a morning meal is the right start, and eating every 4-5 hours will supply regular fuel your body needs. Amazing energy will be found that you never knew you had when you follow this plan.

For most women, 1,200 to 1,400 calories per day are needed to get to that smaller dress size.

For most men, 1,800 to 2,000 calories per day are needed to tighten the belt one hole closer.

Eating three meals a day with a healthy snack works best for most. This regime equates to:

1,200 calories	350 calorie meals with 150 calorie snack
1,400 calories	450 calorie meals with 50 calorie snack
1,600 calories	500 calorie meals with 100 calorie snack
1,800 calories	550 calorie meals with 150 calorie snack

As discussed previously, nutrient rich foods are the best choices. This means put down most of those 100 calorie snack packs, and pick up a fresh fruit, a light yogurt or ½ ounce of nuts. These foods offer more nutrition and more satisfaction.

Think of **a balanced plate with ¼ lean protein, ¼ whole grain, and half vegetables and fruit.** Aim for at least three different colors on your plate. You could be eating delicious meals that look like this:

A simple guide to keep you at **400 calorie meals** is to enjoy 3 ounces of lean protein (150 calories), one whole grain (100 calories) two colorful vegetables (50 calories), one healthy fat (50 calories) and a fresh fruit (50 calories)

HEALTHY TEX-MEX

If it seems difficult to imagine actually preparing and eating these meals, don't worry, you will be guided with helpful tips on planning for the week, grocery shopping, preparing larger amounts and storing until needed, and coming up with new ideas to feed you and your family.

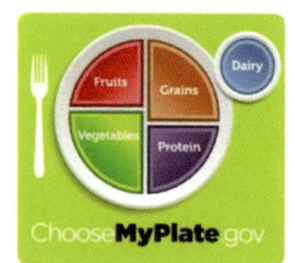

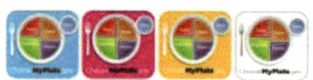

Your physical activity level is just as important as watching the number of calories consumed. Look at physical activity as a necessary part of your life, and don't place the focus on how many calories that activity burns. You can obtain a false sense of negative calorie balance with increased exercise and wind up eating more thus negating the benefits of the activity to your weight loss efforts.

Don't lose hope if you are not a numbers person and do not care to count calories. Understand that if you cut back portions of the foods you are eating now, you can see some weight loss. You can also focus on the powerhouse foods to include in your diet and watch as the other caloric rich choices you used to eat decrease.

Set realistic goals like eating a fresh fruit and a fresh vegetable daily, then increase to 2 and so on. You will soon realize that the chips and fries suddenly decrease, and therefore the calories for the day are decreased.

On occasion you may want your Mom's carne guisada with her homemade flour tortillas. Enjoy and savor the flavors of one and include a big spinach salad with some sliced cucumbers and calories can still be controlled. The danger lies when your favorite food is consumed in larger amounts because you feel you blew it anyway. Just find that balance with lower calorie options, and you will still see that number on the scale go down.

Tortilla Trimmer:

One goal can be to include at least 5 fresh fruit and vegetables per day.

Balancing that seesaw the way you want it to lean takes discipline with calorie control. Every calorie counts that goes into your mouth. The calories you eat in front of people or by yourself, the calories you consume at a table, in your car, in the kitchen cleaning up, or at the movies, the calories in the extra dollop of margarine and the leftover fries from your child- they all count. Start being aware of what is going in, and you will be on your way to successful weight loss.

CALORIES!

Chapter 3 SLIM GEMS

*Success lies in the balance of calories consumed with the calories burned
*Determine your healthy weight
*Estimate the calories your body needs to maintain your weight
*Start with a 250 calorie or 500 calorie reduction per day
*Keep a daily record of what, how much and why you are eating.
*Plan to spend your calorie budget wisely with nutrient rich choices and balance meals including lean protein, whole grain, vegetables and fresh fruit.

Suggested belt reducing goals:

- I will pack my lunch for work Mon-Thurs and choose a restaurant that offers healthy options on Friday.
- I will include a whole grain, two vegetables at lunch instead of avoiding carbohydrates, which will help my afternoon energy low.
- I will keep record of everything I eat and drink by entering everything on myfitnesspal.com or writing it in my food journal
- I will enjoy corn tortilla in place of my two flour tortillas and save 100 calories per day
- I will eat snack pack of popcorn at night instead of chips and save 150 calories.
- I will choose 4 ounces of grilled chicken, lean ground beef, turkey, and fish for lunch and dinner and only allow a fried food on Saturday.
- I will try different light dressings until I find one I enjoy and use a 50-calorie serving on my salad.
- I will cut the habit of a milkshake, and eat a light flavored yogurt.
- This week I will include one calorie controlled meal per day from the South Texas Diet.
- I will cut my avocado in 5 slices and distribute it among the family.
- I will save my favorite restaurant for Sunday morning to enjoy my favorite fluffy pancakes and eggs, but I will not eat the sausage and bacon (that I don't enjoy that much anyways).

CHAPTER 4:
WHAT DO I SEE?

Walk through your home taking inventory. Are there tempting foods on the kitchen counter or in the pantry that you or no one in the house needs to be eating on a regular basis? Are sodas the first thing you see when you open your refrigerator? Surely the freezer has a certain creamy substance that calls out your name every time you open it to get ice.

If this sounds familiar, consider these foods in your belly or better yet on your thighs. There are ways to resist temptation, and you can always work on this, but let's not add to the challenge yet. An important tip to remember is out of sight makes it easier to be out of mind. Better yet **out of the house out of the mouth**. Tempting foods that you tend to over indulge, remove immediately. Once a month, go out for that treat. Take the same look at your work environment or your travel to work. Are there foods you can remove? Or can you arrange your day to avoid seeing those tempting foods?

Tortilla Trimmer:

Out of the house, out of the mouth

Once your surroundings are cleaned up, you can set a plan of action for the foods that you cannot remove and will need to deal with. Write your plan of action in handling the internal thoughts and your outward actions in your journal. Realize the food does not have power over you. You have the control!

Chapter 4: SLIM GEMS

- ⬥ I will chew a piece of gum when cooking to control my nibbling.
- ⬥ I will wash and cut baby carrots, celery and cucumbers to have in a bowl on the top shelf of refrigerator.
- ⬥ I will have a pre-packed healthy snack (see Appendix D) if I get the munchies and avoid walking through the break room at work.
- ⬥ Ice cream being my favorite, I will discard all ice cream from the house and only once a month go out with my family to get a kids scoop of my favorite flavor.
- ⬥ Knowing nuts are so good for me, I will portion 6 walnuts, almonds or cashews in a small baggie for my afternoon snack and not keep the jar of nuts on the counter.

CHAPTER 5:
MASTERING GROCERY SHOPPING AND PORTION CONTROL

Many things in life can sabotage your weight loss efforts with the trip to the grocery store being high on the list. What you buy today will be consumed. So, if a healthy eating plan that helps you lose weight is important to you, don't buy food that will work against your goals.

You might have heard all the tricks to successful grocery shopping, but have you tried them? Make a point to try some of these tips and you will have gained a valuable tool to help with your weight loss efforts.

How to grocery shop successfully

1. Write a list of healthy items and stick to the list. Limit impulsive buying!
2. Careful with snack foods. "It is for the kids" doesn't help your weight loss efforts and many times that food isn't good for them either.
3. Always plan for your shopping trip after a meal.
4. Focus on the perimeter of the store for the lean meats, fruits and vegetables, nonfat dairy and shop the inside isles for whole grains. There may be some isles you do not even go down, and that is okay.
5. Allow time to read nutrition food labels.

Reading labels

Focus on a few things when reading nutrition food labels.

1. Serving size-Is the amount stated the amount you are going to eat? If not you may have to double the numbers given.
2. Calories are important! Is it a side item or is it the main entrée? If you plan for a meal 400-500 calories total then you can better judge how and if that is a good choice.
3. Choose items with less saturated fat and as low as possible of trans fat and include more unsaturated fats.
4. Sodium-is it a side item or main entrée? What else will you be eating with it? Aim for no more than 500-700 mg of sodium per meal.
5. Fiber and sugar are carbohydrates. Generally the more fiber the better and less sugar the better. Aim for at least 3 grams of fiber per serving. The total sugar will be listed including natural sugars like the lactose in dairy and the fructose in fruit. There are 4 grams of sugar in one teaspoon.
6. The ingredient list is helpful to find in descending order the most abundant ingredients. So if sugar is one of the first three ingredients or if different forms of sugar are listed throughout, you can be sure that it is providing too much sugar.

More time is required to make these informed choices, but aren't you and your family worth it! You accomplished an important step in getting healthy foods in your house. Now you have to put it all into action. With your master plan for the week, you can be assured that fruit and vegetables won't wilt away before they are enjoyed, and sodas won't be consumed because there aren't any in the house. Let me remind you of an important point. **You can be eating only healthy foods, but if portion control is not practiced your goals will not be achieved**.

Portion control is the key to weight loss. Keeping a food journal will help you realize how much you are eating and from there you can start cutting back. You may need to weigh and measure cooked foods for a good week to become familiar with proper serving sizes. Use snack size bags to portion foods like whole wheat crackers and nuts.

Tortilla Trimmer:
Tips to help with portion control

- Use a smaller plate.
- Use smaller utensils.
- Serve plates in the kitchen and not at the dinner table.
- Set your fork down between bites.
- Don't be distracted while eating.
- Taking 20 minutes to eat your meal will allow enough time for the brain-stomach connection to register that you have had enough. Eating too quickly doesn't allow the time needed to receive a fullness feeling, and therefore too much food is usually consumed. By taking the time and actually enjoying the flavors of your food, your meal satisfaction can increase and chances for snacking later decrease.

Tortilla Trimmer:
The Many Names of Sugar

- Agave nectar
- brown sugar
- cane sugar
- corn sweetener
- corn syrup
- crystalline fructose
- dextrose
- fructose
- glucose
- high-fructose corn syrup
- honey
- invert sugar
- maltose
- malt syrup
- molasses
- raw sugar
- sucrose

Chapter 5: Slim GEMS

- ◆ I will review the Tips for Grocery Shopping before going to the store.
- ◆ I will cut out the How to Read Labels from the Appendix and bring it with me when grocery shopping.
- ◆ I will use a smaller plate.
- ◆ I will use smaller utensils.
- ◆ I will serve plates in the kitchen and not at the dinner table.
- ◆ I will set my fork down between bites.
- ◆ I won't be distracted while eating.
- ◆ I will take 20 minutes to eat my meals

CHAPTER 6:
EMOTIONAL EATING

Eating to live versus living to eat. What does that look like?

I eat because I actually feel hungry.	Vs.	I eat when I am happy or to celebrate.
		I eat when I am lonely, sad or mad.
		I eat until I finish my plate.
		I eat when I am stressed.
		I eat when I have a craving.
FOOD NOURISHES MY BODY	VS.	I THINK ABOUT FOOD ALL THE TIME.

We all know that hunger is not the only reason we eat. The majority of people use food to deal with their emotions. Emotional eating is eating for reasons other than hunger. If this has become a routine of yours, now is the time to address it.

Celebrate!

Life is full as celebrations as it should be. Food is traditionally the center of those celebrations. Focusing on the people you love and enjoy can bring even more satisfaction than eating unlimited amounts of food. If socializing is not your favorite, you could bring cards or a board game or maybe even all your scrapbooking supplies to teach the younger generation a skill. The idea is to celebrate without over consuming food.

Tortilla Trimmer:

Tips to Eating Socially

- Time your prior meals to arrive to the party without being too hungry.
- Offer to bring a dish. Make something healthy that you will enjoy as well.
- Browse the food options at the party and choose your favorites saving the calories from foods that are not your favorite.
- Choose beverages wisely. Calorie containing beverages do not give you a fullness feeling like most foods and therefore usually lead to excessive calories.
- If you need to be holding something in your hands like everyone else, get a glass of water or sparkling water and garnish with a lime slice.
- Mingle with the guests away from the food area where there is constant nibbling.

Lonely, Sad or Mad

Your emotions of loneliness, sadness or being mad can break havoc on your healthy goals. Developing coping skills to deal with your emotions may require professional help. I would encourage you to seek out this help as soon as possible. Like all things in life, we need a plan. Think through times when you respond with these feelings and write in your journal action steps of how you want to deal with it next time.

Journal Entry

What Happens	What I Feel	My New Action Plan
My spouse is out of town with work all the time.	Lonely	Call my sister over for dinner. Join the Zumba Class at my church.
My coworkers leave me out of the conversations.	Sad	Initiate a walking club at work.
My brothers and sisters do not help with the care of Mom.	Mad	Focus on the quality time with Mom.

Finish Your Plate!

A common excuse is "My parents always made me finish my plate when I was growing up." Your childhood has a lot to do with how you think and your actions, but you can change if it is not helping you reach your goals. The first step is to not allow too much food to be on your plate to start with. This means splitting the meal at a restaurant, serving yourself smaller portions or having to say no thank you at times. If you take a close look at yourself, you may notice a pause during your eating time. You probably have reached this almost full feeling, and if you stop there, you will feel just right after the meal. Take the leftovers for another meal or pass it on to a person in need at the next corner. What a wonderful feeling to help someone who is hungry!

Stressed!

Evaluate the level of stress in your life. If you conclude that stress levels are high, you must put into action steps to decrease the stress in your life. Find the help you need to address a lack of organizational skills if that applies to you. You may find reading a good book, or scripture passages will help calm your nerves or a brisk walk or music. Whatever it is surround yourself with these goods things. Did I mention sleep? Are you getting enough? A lack of sleep can affect your moods, your appetite and your desire to take the time to plan for healthy meals.

> Insanity is doing the same thing, over and over again, but expecting different results.
> Albert Einstein

Cravings!

You will be happy to know that almost everyone has cravings. You are perfectly normal. Maximize your weight loss efforts by accepting the fact that cravings will come, and setting the goal of giving in to these cravings less frequently.

Challenge yourself each week to pass when cravings come knowing that one time a week you will say okay and enjoy a portion. Replacing bad habits with healthy habits like eating only when you are slightly hungry is possible! The first step for you is to determine the reasons why you eat.

Figure out why you are eating by keeping a food journal and including what you ate and what you were feeling at the time. Identify what spurs you to eat and then spend time in planning out what you will do in place of eating to deal with your emotions, habits formed since childhood, and cravings. Let's look at an example:

Tortilla Trimmer:

Steps to overcome cravings

- Identify the foods you crave. Plan for similar foods that are less calories and healthier. Favorite flavored light yogurt in place of ice cream or Carrots with dip made with greek yogurt in place of chips and dip.
- Package smaller portions of the foods you crave. One ounce portion of baked chips in place of eating out of the bag of baked or regular chips.
- Keep the foods that tempt you the most out of hands reach.
- Make a deal with yourself that you will not give in to the craving immediately. Get busy with another activity for 15 minutes and then if you still want it then have a small portion.
- A quick fix is to brush your teeth or chew sugar free mint gum.

My Food Journal Before

	What I Ate	**What was I feeling**	**How did I feel after**
8am	1 c Fiber One 1c skim milk 1 boiled egg	Slightly hungry	Satisfied
2pm	Hamburger Med Fries 16 oz Soda	Stressed about a deadline, very hungry, distracted when eating	Too full, didn't really pay attention when eating
4pm	2 Brownies	Been thinking about the brownies since I saw them in the breakroom this morning. Felt behind on work, doubting was going to be finished by today's deadline	Felt like I blew it! Too many calories
6pm	1 pkg (6) Cheese Crackers	Everyone else went home and I am still working Need a break from work	Wasn't even hungry and I ate
8pm	1c carne guisada ½ c mashed potatoes ½ c corn 2 flour tortillas with butter	No hunger pains but dinner was already prepared	Stuffed and miserable

In this example we can obviously see many areas needing attention. Without this assignment, this person might not have noticed the reasons why she was eating: to get away from working, to try to distract herself of the pressure from work and just because the food was there.

Tortilla Trimmer:

Solutions to Emotional Eating

- Identify actions that help calm nerves during stressful times like listening to soft music, calling a good friend, or sitting in a massage chair.

- Planning for the times of snack attack by packing crunchy vegetables or sugar free jello or even sugar free gum depending on the craving.

- Planning for a healthy snack when mealtime is delayed to prevent getting too hungry.

- When possible sit down with no distractions and enjoy the meal.

After gaining this insight, that day could look like this:

My Food Journal After

	What I Ate	**What was I feeling**	**How did I feel after**
8am	1c Fiber One cereal 1c skim milk 1 boiled egg	slightly hungry, sat down and ate slowly	very satisfied
11:30am	6 oz light yogurt	slightly hungry and know lunch will be delayed	hunger satisfied
2pm	2 corn tortillas 3 oz chicken fajitas Let and tomato 1 c strawberries	slightly hungry, ate slowly	Very satisfied
4pm	Bag of carrots & celery	Everyone eating brownies, just need something to munch on	Felt very good about my choice
6pm	Turned on background music that I love	Stressed about the deadline	Soothing music helped calm my nerves while continuing to work
8pm	½ c carne guisada ½ c mashed potatoes 1 c broccoli 1 c skim milk	Slightly hungry	Satisfied with choices and balance of meal and met my deadline so celebrated by walking to the park with the kids.

Setting realistic goals and working towards them will help you develop a healthy lifestyle. You did not arrive at this point in life overnight so don't expect overnight success.

> The secret about getting ahead is getting started.
>
> Mark Twain

Chapter 6: Slim GEMS

- I will read over the Tips for Eating Socially before going to a family gathering, work function, or any other occasion where eating socially will occur.
- I will write "why" I eat in my food journal to gain a better understanding of my eating habits.
- I will seek ways to handle my emotions without food when I feel sad, mad, or lonely. Even if it means seeking professional help.
- I will follow the Steps to Controlling Cravings to curb my cravings from getting in the way of reaching my goals.
- I will identify actions that help calm nerves during stressful times like listening to soft music, calling a good friend, or sitting in a massage chair.
- I will plan for the times of snack attack by packing crunchy vegetables or sugar free jello or even sugar free gum depending on the craving.
- I will plan for a healthy snack when mealtime is delayed to prevent getting too hungry.
- When possible, I will sit down with no distractions and enjoy the meal.

CHAPTER 7:
WHAT IS FOR DINNER?

Spend some time looking at your week ahead. What activities do you and the family have? Identify the evenings you need quick meals and plan for more convenient healthy choices. For example, on the night you have to take your kids to practice, set out the frozen chicken breast and curry rice from the freezer that you had cooked on the weekend. When you get home, have your older child set the table and your other kiddo toss the spinach salad with light cilantro dressing while you are warming the corn tortillas on the stove and the meat and rice warm in the microwave. In ten minutes you are all sitting down at the table enjoying a delicious well-balanced meal and actually engaging in some good conversation. Even if the whole family can't sit down at the same time, you are providing more satisfying nutritious meals for your family.

You may have experienced hesitations from your kids to eat certain new things in the past. Don't give up! Include them in the shopping and preparation, and you may see a renewed interest. There are many benefits found when you involve your kids and have regular family meals. Think about the great memories you are creating. The children will learn over time how to follow a recipe, food safety and that it is actually fun to create delicious food.

After looking at the schedule for the upcoming activities you can plan what meals will be best for each day, and therefore shop for those foods. Utilizing the days you have more time to prepare foods and store in the freezer and to prewash fruit and vegetables to have them visible and ready to eat, which will allow you to feed your family in a healthier way.

Life Before the South Texas Slim Down

You are driving home from work and need to pick up your two kids, and you have about 90 minutes before you are expected at the basketball practice. You don't know what is at home, so you swing by a fast food place and pick up three meals. The kids eat in the car, and you wait until you get home and eat alone in front of the TV. The kids go to their rooms and play video games and when it is time to leave you all get in the car.

Life After the South Texas Slim Down

Before you leave for work in the morning, you place the chicken fajitas and whole beans out of the freezer into the refrigerator. You pick up the kids and talk about the day on the way home. When you get home you ask the older kids to set the table while you peel two oranges and wash the cherry tomatoes. Meanwhile you warm up the fajitas, beans and corn tortillas. Within ten minutes you all are sitting down at the dinner table enjoying a delicious healthy meal together. You are out the door feeling great and ready for the evening activity.

Putting some thought into your choices will allow for less stress on busy days. Consider getting the measuring cups and scales out to teach your children portion control. Weigh out the chicken breast and the ground lean meat and account for 3-4 ounces per person and place it in a freezer bag ready to go for the next meal. Measure out the rice after it is cooked and see what one half cup looks like. Place the two cups of rice for the four of you, and you can be sure that everyone will get the healthy amount.

Utilizing slow cookers and inside mini grills can also allow for delicious healthy convenient meals. Boneless pork chops or fresh fish takes only minutes on the inside grill that cook top and bottom at the same time. Slow cookers you can put meals together in the morning and come home to a meal ready to eat.

The time you invest in planning your family meals will allow for healthier meals, appropriate portions, and quality time together that you will never regret. **It may be difficult to start this process, but like everything else it gets easier once the new habits are established.**

Use the following form to plan your meals for the week based on your schedule identifying heavy work days, busy afternoon activities for the kids, family celebrations and anything else that adds to your day.

HEALTHY TEX-MEX

An example of enjoying healthy meals with a busy week:

Sunday	Monday	Tuesday	Wednesday
9-10am church Huevos Rancheros banana/straw berries	7am son's football practice Light yogurt, peach and walnuts Take fish out of freezer for tonight	Raisin bran with skim milk Pack work snack and sides for sandwich at track meet	6:30am home exercise Boiled egg, ww toast, skim milk, plum Take gr. Turkey out of freezer and pack lunch
11-1pm lunch with abuelo & abuela choose grilled snapper with veggies Grocery shop Make brwn rice w/ corn & beans and freeze Marinate chick fajitas Make green salsa for the week	Extra busy at work Pack a lunch chicken fajitas over salad, ww crackers and grapes	Out for lunch Choose the caldo with corn tortilla Pack an apple and string chz for snack	Packed lunch Lime Roasted Chicken w/ Green salsa Rice w/corn, beans and sliced cucumbers
Family meal Chick Fajitas, Corn tort, spinach salad, light dressing Fresh corn on the cob, mango slices	5-6 Drum practice Gr fish tacos frozen veg mix 30 minute walk	5-8pm Go to the track meet Pick up sub sandwiches With prepacked sides of veggies and dip, ww pretzels Take cooked chicken legs out of freezer for pack lunch	Walk to the park before dinner Turkey chili w/ salad

Thursday	Friday	Saturday
7am son's football practice Oatmeal with milk and cranberries Take out cooked grnd beef from freezer. Pack lunch	7am Early shift at work Whole grain cereal, skim milk, almonds Take out pork chops from freezer	7-12pm garage sale Egg/cheese taco w/ green salsa Snack on apple slices
Doctor's apt at lunch Packed lunch of ww bread, turkey, l&t, mustard, celery, light yogurt	Packed lunch of lettuce wraps with watermelon	12-4pm BBQ volunteer BBQ chicken, green beans and pinto beans Take home BBQ plates for dinner
7-9pm PTA Lettuce wrap, rice w/ corn, beans, zucchini w/ tomatoes Pack lunch for tomorrow	Family meal to celebrate birthday Pork chop w/ corn relish, sweet potatoes, green beans with tomatoes Angel Food cake w/ strawberries Family game of basketball	7-10pm Hooks baseball game BBQ plate Take large bottle of water, get up every hour and walk for 20 minutes

There may be times that you are not able to stick to the original plan but at least you are prepared with healthy food options for you and your family that will help you reach your goal of losing weight the healthy way.

Chapter 7: Slim GEMS

- ♦ I will involve the kids in meal planning and preparation.
- ♦ I will plan my meals for a week using the Meal Planner chart in Appendix C.
- ♦ I won't give up if I can't stick to the original plan. The next day I will continue using my meal plan.

CHAPTER 8:
RECIPES

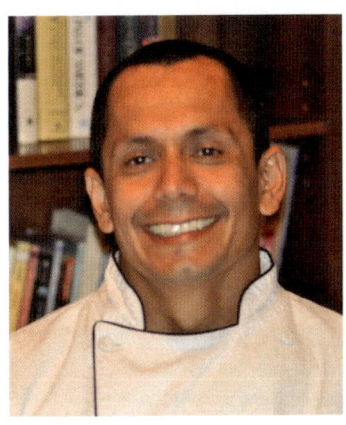

Mario Mantilla received his Bachelor Degree of Science in Food Science from La Universidad de la Salle in Colombia, South America. After running his own restaurant in Colombia, he moved to Corpus Christi, Texas where he trained in the Culinary Art program at both Del Mar Community College and at the Culinary Institute of America in San Antonio. Mario was the head chef at the locally famous seafood restaurant, The Yardarm, in Corpus Christi for fourteen years. He enjoyed the culinary challenge of creating healthy and flavorful traditional South-Texas cuisine; "I sincerely hope that you will enjoy discovering the unique flavors of South Texas in the dishes that follow."

How to use the recipe section of the book

We have created these tasty recipes to maintain the flavors of South Texas Cuisine. Do not feel limited to eating only these recipes; rather, use these recipes when you feel like having some of your favorite Tex-Mex cuisine. You'll be surprised how our recipes are healthier, yet maintain the great flavor we all love.

Pay special attention to the serving sizes listed on most recipes. You will not see any changes in your waistline if you eat too large of a portion. Rather, serve yourself a single serving and eat slowly, savoring each flavorful bite.

We designed the recipes to **help save you time preparing food throughout the week**, but in order to save time; you WILL have to do some planning. The SIDES section is full of recipes that the MEALS section require. So, look through the main dishes, and look at the ingredient list- there you will see in a **green text** the side dish that needs to be prepared in advance to make the meal. I recommend selecting a few main dishes for the week that require the same side dishes. For example, **Huevos Rancheros**, **Turkey and Corn Quesidillas**, **Meatloaf**, and **Blackbean and Butternut Tacos** require you make the **Roasted Tomato Oregano Chunky Sauce** and the **Refried Beans**. So, on the weekend when you grocery shop, prepare the Roasted Tomato Oregano Chunky Sauce and the Refried Beans, and you will have them on-hand during the week when you prepare the four meals. A little planning and time upfront will make huge differences on your overall health and well-being.

We definitely prefer preparing foods with fresh ingredients (fresh tomatoes vs. canned tomatoes, home-made refried beans vs. canned refried beans, ect…) However, sometimes life just gets too busy to allow the extra time, so we have included some shortcuts in the margins titled "Time Crunch?" to help save you time. Many of the tips can be used to save time with multiple recipes- they are not limited to the recipes by their sides. When you do have the time, make the foods from scratch- they are healthier and tastier; but don't feel guilty on those weeks where you just don't have enough time.

Tbs- tablespoon

tsp- teaspoon

C- cup

oz- ounce

RECIPES

SIDES

SOUTH TEXAS SLIM DOWN SPECIAL SEASONING

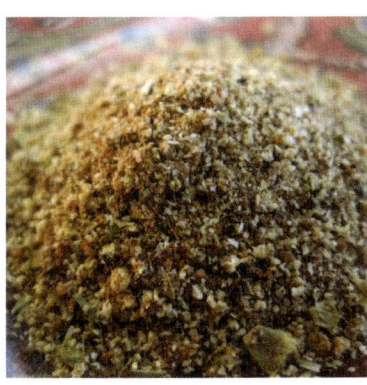

1. Mix all the ingredients in a bowl.
2. Spoon mixture into a tightly closed container and label. Store in a cool, dry place. Use within 6 months.

Saucy Suggestion:
- Use for meatloaf, burgers, tacos, tomato sauce, casseroles, dips, and any dish you like.

10 calories; 2g carb; .3g pro; .2g fat; 0g sat'd; 0g trans; 0mg chol; .5g fiber; .5g sugar; 75mg Na

Makes: 9 servings
Serving size 1 tsp

1Tbs	ground onions
2tsp	chili powder
1tsp	garlic powder
1tsp	cornstarch
1tsp	cumin
½tsp	cayenne pepper
1tsp	dry oregano
½ tsp	black pepper
¼ tsp	sea salt

Recipes that Require this Side:

Zuchini and Tomatoes pg 60
Chicken Fajitas pg 70
Turkey Chili pg 71
Chilaquiles pg 74
Lime-Roasted Chicken with Green Salsa pg 75
Chalupas pg 76
Lettuce Wraps pg 80
Pasta with Ground Beef and Tomato Sauce pg 81
Grilled Fish Tacos pg 82
Pork Chops with Corn-Bell Pepper Relish pg 84
Refried Bean and Butternut Tacos pg 85
Refried Bean Burgers with Guacamole pg 87

GUACAMOLE

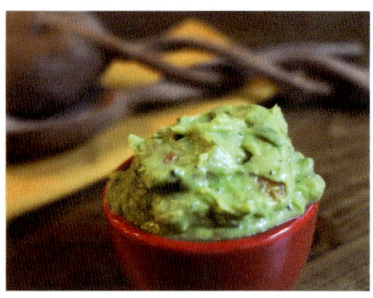

Prep time: 30 minutes
Makes 20 servings
(Serving size: ¼ cup)

3	ripe medium avocados
¼ C	red onion minced
3	garlic cloves, peeled
½ C	fresh cilantro, chopped
1	ripe tomato, diced
1	bunch green onion, sliced
2 Tbs	lime juice
2 T	red wine vinegar
½ tsp	chili powder
2 tsp	salt
1 tsp	black pepper

1. Heat small skillet on low heat with olive oil, sauté garlic cloves; cook, turning occasionally, until soft and blackened in spots. Cool. Finely chop.
2. In a large bowl, add sautéed chopped garlic, cilantro, red onion, tomatoes, green onions, lime juice, vinegar, oil, and scoop avocado. Coarsely mash everything together until desired texture.
3. Add chili powder, salt, and black pepper. Transfer to a serving bowl and place plastic wrap directly on the surface of the guacamole (to prevent browning). * Tip: - Refrigerate up to 3 days.

Saucy Suggestion:
- Next time add some plain yogurt, light sour cream or light mayonnaise and half-half to create a new dressing to serve with chicken, fish, green salad or pasta (for 1C of guacamole; add 2T yogurt, 2T sour cream or mayonnaise and 1T half-half, and adjust the flavor with salt and pepper).
- You can also serve this as a dip or sandwich filling.

67 calories; 4g carb; 1g pro; 6g fat; 1g sat'd; 0g trans; 0 mg chol; 2.3g fiber; .7g sugar; 63mg Na

Recipes that Require this Side:

Huevos Rancheros pg 66

Omelets pg 67

Huevos Rancheros Verdes pg 68

Turkey and Pepper Burritos pg 69

Grilled Fish Tacos pg 80

Refried Bean Burgers with Guacamole pg 87

Refried Bean Cakes with Guacamole Dressing pg 88

REFRIED BEANS

Prep time: 1:30 – 2 hours
Makes 16 servings (serving size: ½ cup)

1	onion, peeled and halved
3C	dry pinto beans, rinsed
½	fresh jalapeño pepper, seeded, chopped
2Tbs	cloves garlic, minced
5tsp	sea salt
1 ¾ tsp	fresh ground black pepper
⅛ tsp	ground cumin
9C	water or as needed

1. Rinse beans, and soak overnight.
2. Place the onion, beans, pepper, garlic, sea salt, ground black pepper, and cumin into a pot. Pour in the water, and stir to combine. Cook on high until boiling, then reduce the heat (set on medium) and simmer until the beans are soft, more or less 1 hour and 30 minutes to 2 hours, adding more water as needed.
3. Once the beans have cooked, strain them reserving liquid. Mash the beans with a potato masher; adding the reserved water as needed to reach desired consistency.

144 calories; 27g carb; 9g pro; .5g fat; 0g sat'd; 0g trans; 0mg chol; 6.3g fiber; 2 g sugar; 788mg Na

---

Recipes that Require this Side:

Huevos Rancheros pg 66

Omelets pg 67

Huevos Rancheros Verdes pg 68

Chalupas pg 76

Refried Bean and Butternut Tacos pg 85

Refried Bean Burgers with Guacamole pg 87

Refried Bean Cakes with Guacamole Dressing pg 88

⏲ Time Crunch?

Buy sodium-reduced canned refried beans, but know you will be sacrificing flavor

ROASTED TOMATO OREGANO CHUNKY SAUCE

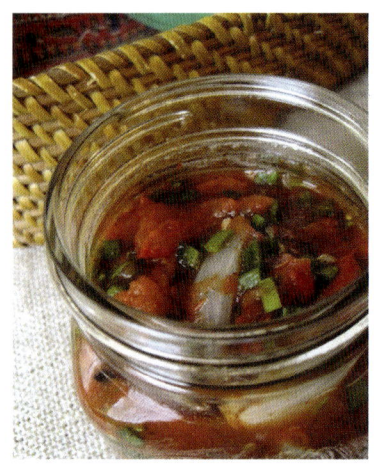

Prep time: 30 minutes
Makes 8 servings (serving size: ½ cup)

6	plum tomatoes
1	small yellow onion, quartered
1	garlic clove
2	jalapeno, chopped
1	bunch green onion, only green part, sliced
3 Tbs	fresh oregano, chopped
½ tsp	ground cumin
½ C	water
1 tsp	salt
1 Tbs	chili powder
2 Tbs	Lime juice

1. Preheat oven to 420
2. Use a baking pan and add tomatoes, yellow onion, and garlic. Roast until brown and soft, about 20 minutes.
3. Transfer roasted mixture to a bowl and smash together with remaining ingredients. Chill, covered.

Saucy Suggestion:
- Make the sauce ahead of time to develop more flavor.
- Puree sauce and try it with all your favorite food.
- *Refrigerate for up to 5 days or freeze in an airtight container for up to 6 months.*

30 calories, 6.6g carb, 1.3g pro, .4g fat, 0g sat'd, 0g trans, 0mg chol, 2g fiber, 3.3 g sugar, 96mg Na

---

Recipes that Require this Side:

Huevos Rancheros pg 66

Turkey and Corn Quesadillas pg#

Meatloaf pg 72

Stuffed Pepper with Mango Salsa pg 78

Lettuce Wraps pg 80

Chorizo Migas pg 79

Pasta with Ground Beef and Tomato Sauce pg 81

Refried Bean and Butternut Tacos pg 85

GREEN SALSA

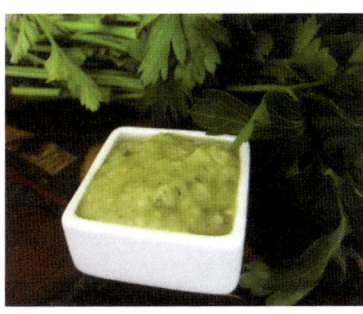

Prep time: 30 minutes
Makes 16 servings (serving size: ¼ cup)

1Lb	tomatillos, quartered
3	garlic cloves
1	jalapeno
2	shallots
1	red onion, sliced
2	ripe avocado, sliced
1	bunch Cilantro, chopped
2 Tbsp	lime juice
½ tsp	cumin
1 ½ C	water depending on the thickness desired
1tsp	salt
½ tsp	ground black pepper

1. Remove husks from tomatillos and rinse well. Cook the tomatillos in the boiling water until soft. Drain and reserve some water (1 C).
2. Toast garlic, jalapeno, shallots, and onion in a dry skillet over medium heat, turning occasionally, until browned and soft.
3. Combine the tomatillos, garlic mixture, lime juice, and avocados in a food processor. Process until smooth (Add some of the reserved water to reach desired consistency). Stir in cilantro, cumin, salt and pepper.

Saucy Suggestion:
The salsa can be prepared ahead of time. Cover and refrigerate for up to 5 days.

56 calories, 5g carb, 1g pro, 4g fat, .6g sat'd, 0g trans, 0mg chol, 2.6 g fiber, 1.7g sugar, 78 mg Na

Recipes that Require this Side:

Huevos Rancheros Verdes pg 68

Turkey and Pepper Burritos pg 69

Chicken Fajitas pg 70

Tortilla Chip-Crusted Chicken with Green Salsa pg 73

Chilaquiles pg 74

Lime-Roasted Chicken with Green Salsa pg 75

Chalupas pg 76

Chorizo Migas pg 79

Refried Bean and Butternut Tacos pg 85

COLESLAW

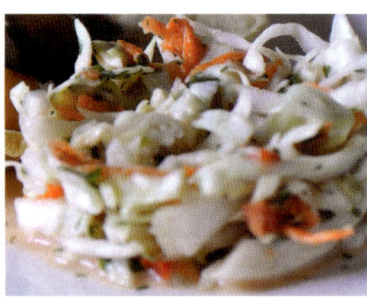

Prep time: 20 minutes
Makes 8 servings (serving size: 1/3 cup)

1	head thinly sliced green cabbage
1 C	carrots, peeled and grated
⅓ C	cilantro, chopped
¾ C	kernel corn, from can
¾ C	red bell pepper, chopped
2 Tbs	canola oil
⅓ C	fat-free mayonnaise
¼ C	rice vinegar
1 T	lime juice
2 tsp	honey
¼ tsp	ground cumin
¼ tsp	Salt

1. In a small bowl, stir together mayonnaise, lime juice, vinegar, honey, and cumin.
2. In a large bowl place cabbage, carrots, corn, red bell pepper, and cilantro. Pour mayonnaise mixture over cabbage mixture. Toss lightly to coat.
3. Serve or cover and chill up to 4 days.

89 calories, 12.6g carb, 1.5 g pro, 4 g fat, 6g sat'd, 0g trans, 1mg chol, 2.8g fiber, 6.2g sugar, 181 mg Na

Recipes that Require this Side:

Grilled Fish Tacos pg 82

Refried Bean and Butternut Tacos pg 85

🕐 Time Crunch?

Buy a package of coleslaw in the produce department, use the chopped mixture and throw away the sauce packet. Also, purchase grated carrots.

CORN AND BELL PEPPER RELISH

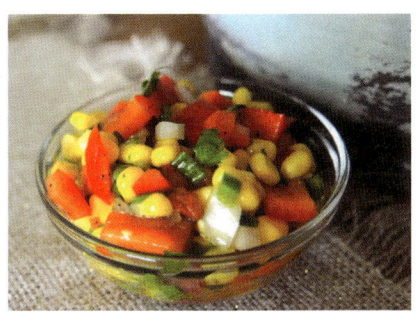

Prep time: 20 minutes
Makes 8 servings (serving size: ¼ cup)

½ C	ripe tomatoes, diced
¼ C	sweet onion, chopped
2	jalapeno, diced
2 C	thawed frozen corn kernels
2	stalks green onion, chopped
2	red bell pepper, diced
2 Tbs	lime juice
4 Tbs	extra virgin olive oil
3 Tbs	white wine vinegar
1 Tbs	honey
2 tsp	fresh cilantro, chopped
1 tsp	salt
½ tsp	ground black pepper

1. In a big bowl, gently stir tomatoes, onion, jalapeno, corn, bell pepper, and cilantro. Then add all the liquids and toss well.
2. Season with salt and pepper.
3. Chill up to 5 days.

Saucy Suggestion:
This relish is a great side to almost any dish! It also makes a great side to bring to a party.

131 calories, 15g carb, 2g pro, 7.4 g fat, 1g sat'd, 0g trans, 0mg chol, 1.8 g fiber, 5.3 g sugar, 77mg Na

Recipes that Require this Side:

Pork Chops and Corn-Bell Pepper Relish pg 84

MANGO SALSA

Prep time: 20 minutes
Makes 16 servings (serving size: ¼ cup)

2C	mangoes, chopped
1C	red bell pepper, diced
⅓ C	red onion, diced
1	jalapeño, diced
¼ C	fresh cilantro leaves, chopped
1C	green onion (green part only) sliced
2Tbs	lime juice
1tsp	garlic powder
pinch	chili powder
1tsp	salt
½ tsp	black pepper

1. In a bowl mix all the ingredients. Cover and chill for 1 hour before serving.
2. Refrigerate for up to 3 days.

Saucy Suggestion:
This salsa is easy to make and perfect with fish or to top fish tacos.

19 cal, 5g carb, .4g pro, .1g fat, 0g sat'd, 0g trans, 0mg chol, .7g fiber, 4g sugar, 38mg Na

Recipes that Require this Side:

Stuffed Peppers with Mango Salsa pg 78

Grilled Fish Tacos pg 82

CILANTRO DRESSING

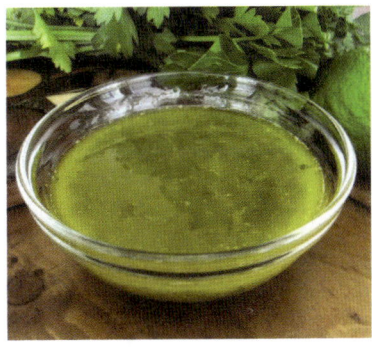

Prep time: 15 minutes
Makes 2 cups (serving size: 1 Tbsp)

3/4 C	fresh cilantro, chopped
1-2	garlic cloves
¼	small yellow onion, sautéed until brown
1 Tbs	minced seed jalapeño
3-4 Tbs	white wine vinegar
2 Tbs	lime juice
1 ½ Tbs	honey
1 C	olive oil
¼ tsp	cumin
1.5 tsp	salt
½ tsp	fresh ground black pepper

1. In skillet, heat 1tsp oil and add onion and sauté until browned.
2. In a food processor, combine the cilantro, garlic, sautéed onion, jalapeno, white vinegar, and lime juice. Process until chopped finely.
3. Add the remainder of the oil with the motor running and blend until almost smooth.
4. Stir in cumin, salt, and black pepper. Cover, and chill for up to 5 days.
5. Before serving, bring to room temperature; and whisk.

Saucy Suggestion:
- You can use this dressing with any salad or to marinade chicken and fish.
- Add ½ cup plain yogurt, plain Greek yogurt or buttermilk for a creamy version of the dressing (just note that this will change the nutrition information for the recipe).

93 calories, 1g carb, .1g pro, 10g fat, 1.4g sat'd, 0 g trans, 0mg chol, .1g fiber, .6g sugar, 110mg Na

JICAMA, MANGO, AND PINEAPPPLE SALSA

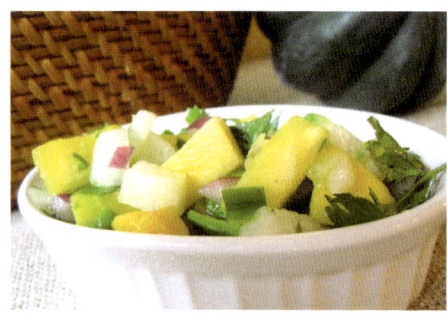

1. In a bowl, toss together all the ingredients. Made ahead to blend the flavors and chill covered.

Saucy Suggestion:
- Use as a side dish, filling, or with grilled fish.

76 calories, 11g carb, 1g pro, 3.8g fat, .6g sat'd, 0g trans, 0 mg chol, 2.8g fiber, 7.5 g sugar, 76 mg Na

Prep time: 15 minutes
Makes 16 servings (serving size ¼ cup)

1C	jicama, diced
1 ¾ C	mangos, diced
1 ¾ C	pineapple, diced
1	ripe avocados, chopped
¼ C	red onion, chopped
½ C	cilantro, chopped
1	small jalapeno, chopped with seeds or without
2 Tbs	orange juice
1 Tbs	honey
½ tsp	salt

⏱ Time Crunch?
Buy the canned diced fruit, but be sure to avoid the syrup added mixtures, and rinse the fruits before using.

MANGO AND ROASTED TOMATO SAUCE

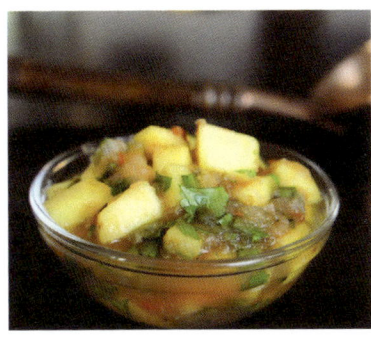

Prep time: 30 minutes
Makes 12 servings (serving size: ¼ cup)

1	ripe mangos, chopped
1	small sweet onion, diced
1	clove garlic
1	green onion, chopped
¼ C	fresh cilantro
¼ C	lime juice
2 Tbs	brown sugar
2	plum tomatoes
1	jalapeno, minced
1 tsp	salt
1 Tbs	hot sauce (optional)

1. Preheat oven to 400
2. Quarter tomatoes and place in a baking pan with onions, garlic, cilantro, and jalapeno. Transfer to the oven and roast for 15 minutes.
3. Chop mango.
4. In a blender puree roasted tomatoes, lime juice, sugar, and hot sauce until smooth.
5. In a bowl, stir together pureed tomato mixture, mango, and salt.

Saucy Suggestion:
- Serve on fish, pork tenderloin, or chicken.
- To improve the flavor made the sauce one day ahead and chilled covered.

74 calories, 17g carb, 2g pro, .3g fat, 0g sat'd, 0g trans, 0mg chol, 1.5g fiber, 8.4 g sugar, 106mg Na

⏲ Time Crunch?
Buy the jarred mangos and chop the slices. And, buy the pre-chopped tomatoes, jalapenos, green onion and cilantro.

GREEN BEANS WITH BASIL AND TOMATOES

Prep time: 20 minutes
Makes 4 servings

1 Tbs	canola oil
½	yellow onion, sliced
1	garlic, minced
¼ tsp	cayenne
1 Lb	green beans, trimmed
2 C	tomatoes, diced
½ tsp	salt
¼ tsp	ground black pepper
2 Tbs	basil, chopped

1. In a saucepan, boil salted water and add beans; cook until tender but crispy, about 7 minutes. Then, transfer to ice water and let rest for few minutes. Drain, set aside.
2. In a skillet, heat oil and add onion, sauté until soft. Add garlic, cayenne pepper, and black pepper; cook for 2 minutes. Add green beans and cook for 2 minutes.
3. Add tomatoes and bring to a boil. Turn down the heat and simmer on low until greens are warm. Sprinkle with chopped basil before serving.

97 calories, 15 g carb, 3 g pro, 4 g fat, .3 g sat'd, 0 trans, 0 chol, 5 g fiber, 160 mg Na

🕐 Time Crunch?
Buy frozen Green Beans

GREEN SALAD

Prep time: 5 minutes
Makes 4 servings

12 Oz	fresh spinach or spring mix
1	tomato, chopped
½ C	red onion, thinly sliced
½	avocado, sliced
⅓ C	**Cilantro Dressing, see pg 55**

1. In a large bowl, combine all the ingredients except the dressing. Drizzle with 1 Tbsp dressing and toss to coat. Serve immediately.

136 calories, 9 g carb, 4 g pro, 11 g fat, 1.5 g sat'd, 0 trans, 0 chol, 4 g fiber, 145 mg Na

ZUCCHINI AND TOMATOES

Prep time: 20 minutes
Makes 8 servings

2 Tbs	canola oil
1	yellow onion, chopped
2	clove garlics, minced
1	can diced tomatoes, no salt added
1 tsp	salt
½ tsp	ground black pepper
5	zucchini, slices
3 Tbs	lemon juice
1 tsp	**Seasoning, see pg 47**

1. Heat oil in a skillet, add onions and sauté for 3 minutes. Add garlic and cook for 1 minute. Stir in tomatoes, salt, and pepper and bring mixture to a boil.
2. Add zucchini and cook for 5 minutes. Drizzle with the lemon juice and serve.

72 calories, 9g carb, 2g pro, 4g fat, .4g sat'd, 0 trans, 0 chol, 2g fiber, 162mg Na

CILANTRO RICE

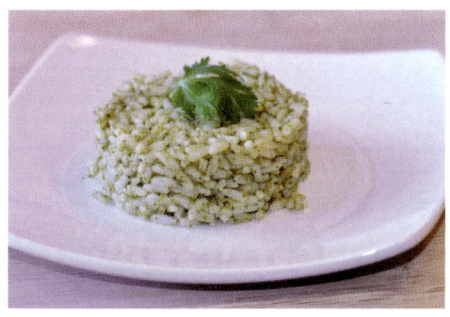

Prep time: 45 minutes
Makes 8 servings
(serving size: ½ cup)

1C	brown rice
2C	water
½	bunch cilantro
½C	white onion, chopped
¼C	green onion, chopped
1 ½ Tbs	jalapeno, chopped
1 ½ Tbs	lime juice
1 Tbs	olive oil
1 tsp	salt
½ tsp	fresh ground black pepper

1. In a blender, puree cilantro, onion, scallions, jalapenos, lime juice, and water until smooth. Add salt and pepper; set aside.
2. In a saucepan, heat oil, add the rice and fry until lightly browned.
3. Add cilantro mixture to browned rice and bring to a boil. Reduce heat to medium-low, cover and simmer for about 35 minutes. Remove from heat, and let stand for 10 minutes. Fluff rice with a fork and add salt and black pepper.

100 cal, 19g carb, 1.7g pro, 2g fat, .3g sat'd, 0g trans, 0mg chol, 1g fiber, 1.4g sugar, 150mg Na

YELLOW RICE

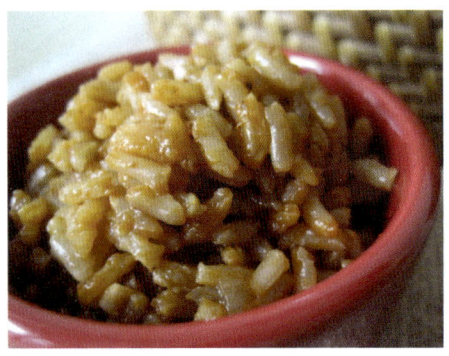

Prep time: 45 minutes
Makes 8 servings (serving size: ½ cup)

2 Tbs	olive oil
1	medium onion, chopped
1	clove of garlic, minced
1 C	brown rice
2 C	chicken broth, low-sodium
1 Tbs	tomato paste
Pinch	achiote powder
Pinch	oregano
1 tsp	salt
½ tsp	fresh ground black pepper

1. In a saucepan, heat olive oil, then add onion and garlic. Cook until onions are tender. Add rice and cook until the rice is browned. Stir in broth, tomato paste, achiote, and oregano.
2. Bring mixture to a boil, reduce heat to medium–low and cover, simmering for 35 minutes. Remove from heat and let sit for 10 minutes. Fluff with a fork and add salt and black pepper.

145 cal, 24g carb, 3.4g pro, 4g fat, .6g sat'd, 0g trans, 0mg chol, 1g fiber, 2.4g sugar, 183mg Na

BROWN RICE

Prep time: 40 minutes
Makes 8 servings
(serving size: ½ cup)

1 Tbs	canola oil
½ C	yellow onion, chopped
1	bay leaf
¼ tsp	dried thyme
Pinch of white pepper	
1 C	brown rice
2 ½ C	chicken broth, low-sodium
1 tsp	salt
½ tsp	ground black pepper

1. In a saucepan, heat oil over medium heat. Add onion and bay leaf, sauté for about 3 minutes. Stir in white pepper and thyme.
2. Add rice; stir for 2 minutes.
3. Add broth and bring to boil.
4. Reduce the heat to medium-low, cover and simmer about 35 minutes. Discard bay leaf, and fluff with a fork adding salt and black pepper.

105 cal, 18g carb, 2.6g pro, 2.4g fat, .3g sat'd, 0g trans, 0mg chol, .7g fiber, 1g sugar, 20mg Na

CURRIED BROWN RICE

Prep time: 30 minutes
Makes 8 servings
(serving size: ½ cup)

1C	brown rice
½C	vermicelli, spaghetti
¼C	chopped almonds
¼C	raisins
1Tbs	yellow curry
¼C	green onion, slice
1tsp	salt
½ tsp	fresh ground black pepper

1. Cook rice according to the instructions in the box. Let rest for 10 minutes
2. In a skillet with 1 Tbsp of canola oil, fry spaghetti until crispy and browned. Stirring constantly.
3. Mix rice with spaghetti, almonds, raisins, curry, green onion, salt and pepper.

149 cal, 28g carb, 3.7g pro, 3g fat, .3g sat'd, 0g trans, 0mg chol, 2.3g fiber, 3g sugar, 177mg Na

Time Crunch?
Skip the vermicelli for this dish

RICE WITH CORN AND BEAN

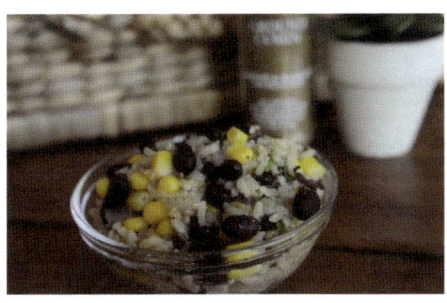

Prep time: 30 minutes
Makes 8 servings (serving size: ½ cup)

2.5–3C	water
½C	yellow onion, minced
1	clove garlic, minced
¾C	thawed, frozen corn
1tsp	ground cumin
½tsp	ground coriander seeds
1C	brown rice
½C	canned black beans, rinsed and drained
2 Tbs	fresh cilantro, chopped
1Tbs	lime juice
1 tsp	salt
½ tsp	ground black pepper

1. In a saucepan, bring water to a boil with garlic, onion, cumin, and coriander seeds. Stir in rice and cook at medium-low heat, covered for 35 minutes. Stir in corn and simmer on low for 10 minutes. Fluff mixture.
2. Rinse and drain black beans. Stir beans into rice with cilantro, lime juice, salt, and black pepper.

124 cal, 26g carb, 3.4g pro, 1g fat, .2g sat'd, 0g trans, 0mg chol, 2.4 g fiber, 1g sugar, 28mg Na

EGGS

HUEVOS RANCHEROS

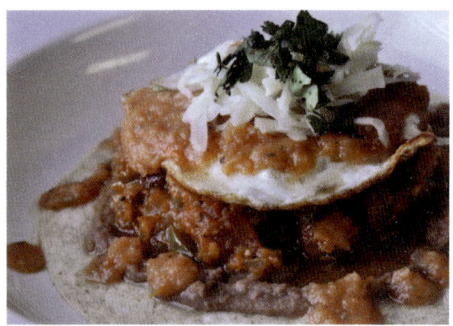

Prep time: 30 minutes
Makes 8 servings

½ Tbs	canola oil
1 C	onion, chopped
½ C	green bell pepper, chopped
2	cloves garlic, minced
1 C	tomatoes, diced reserved liquid
1 C	Roasted Tomato Oregano Chunky Sauce, see page 50
2 C	Refried Beans, warmed, see page 49
	Cooking spray
8	large eggs
8	whole-wheat tortillas
½ C	reduced fat jack cheese
¼½ C	fresh cilantro, chopped

1. In a saucepan, heat oil and add onions, bell peppers, and garlic; sauté until soft. Add the tomatoes and Roasted Tomato Oregano Chunky Sauce; bring to a boil. Reduce heat. Simmer on low until slightly thick. Remove from heat; stir in cilantro. Set aside.
2. Meanwhile, heat skillet with cooking spray. Fry eggs until desired degree of doneness.
3. Heat refried beans in microwave or on stove.
4. Warm tortillas in a skillet or the oven. Divide the beans among them, and top with a fried egg, some tomato sauce and cheese. Sprinkle cilantro for garnish.

Saucy Suggestion:
more flavor, you can serve with Guacamole, see page 48.

341 cal, 51g carb, 19g pro, 8g fat, 3g sat'd, 0g trans, 215mg chol, 8g fiber, 5g sugar, 573mg Na

> ⏲ **Time Crunch?**
>
> Don't have time for all the steps, then just use the Chunky Tomato Oregano Chunky Sauce for the Huevos Rancheros instead of making the tomato and vegetable mixture.

OMELETS

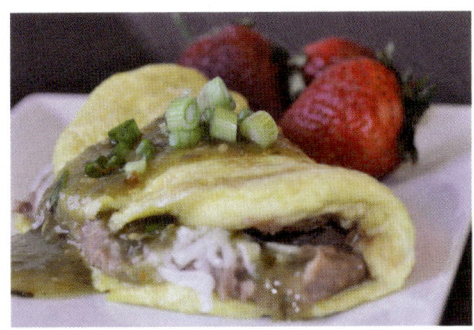

Prep time: 30 minutes
Makes 4 servings

2 tsp canola oil, used ½ tsp per omelet
½ C **Refried Beans see page 49**
4 egg whites
2 eggs
2 Tbs fat-free milk
¼ tsp black pepper
⅓ C reduced fat jack cheese
½ C **Green Salsa, see page 51**
4 Tbs green onion, minced

1. Warm up refried beans in microwave or on the stove. Set aside, and keep warm.
2. In a bowl, combine egg whites, eggs, and milk; stir well. Heat oil in a small skillet over medium high heat. Pour half of the egg mixture into pan. Cook; flip omelet. Spread refried bean onto half of omelet. Sprinkle with cheese. Carefully spread with a spatula. Fold in half. Cook. Slide onto a plate. Spoon some of the **Green Salsa** and scallions. Repeat procedure with remaining ingredients. Serve.

Saucy Suggestion:
- For more flavor, you can serve with Guacamole, see page 48.

169 cal, 11g carb, 12g pro, 9g fat, 3g sat'd, 0g trans, 99mg chol, 3g fiber, 2g sugar, 228mg Na

HUEVOS RANCHEROS VERDES

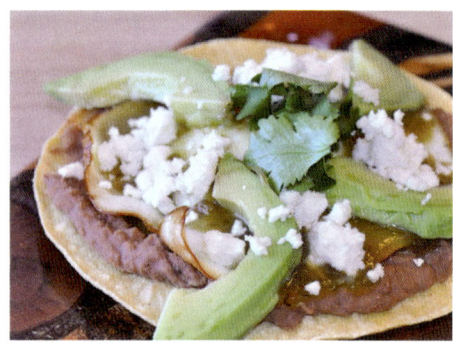

Prep time: 30 minutes
Makes 4 servings

2tsp canola oil
8   corn tortillas
24   eggs
1C   **Refried Beans, warm, see page 49**
½ C   **Green Salsa, see page 51**
½   avocado, sliced
¼ C   feta cheese, crumbled
1 handful sprigs cilantro

1. Warm refried beans in microwave or on stove.
2. Heat oil in a skillet, and add tortillas; toast and set aside. Add a little more oil to the same skillet, and fry eggs sunny side up or until desired doneness.
3. Place a tortilla on each plate and top with the beans followed by the **Green Salsa**, eggs, add more **Green Salsa**, cheese, avocados and cilantro.

Saucy Suggestion:
꙳ For more flavor, you can serve with Guacamole, see page 48.

362cal, 40g carb, 16g pro, 16g fat, 4g sat'd, 0g trans, 194mg chol, 9g fiber, 3g sugar, 324 mg Na

POULTRY

TURKEY AND PEPPER BURRITOS

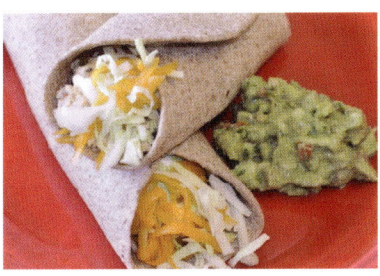

Prep time: 40 minutes
Makes 12 servings

1	medium white onion, chopped
1 Tbs	canola oil
2	cloves garlic, minced
2	red bell pepper, diced
½ 1	yellow bell pepper, diced
1	green bell pepper, diced
1 Tbs	cumin
2 Tbs	dried oregano
4 C	shredded cooked 93% lean turkey
2 tsp	salt
1 tsp	ground black pepper
12	whole wheat tortillas
1 ½ C	low-fat cheddar cheese, shredded
⅓ C	fat free cream cheese
3 C	shredded green cabbage

1. In a large skillet heat oil, and sauté onion until translucent. Stir in garlic, peppers, cumin, and oregano and sauté another 5 minutes. Simmer until the onions are very soft.
2. Stir in turkey and continue cooking until the mixture is heated through.
3. Heat up a skillet on medium-high heat, warm tortillas.
4. Spoon mixture among tortillas. Top each with cheeses and cabbage, roll into burritos and serve.

Saucy Suggestion:
- Serve with **Guacamole or Green Salsa. See pages 48 and 51.**
- Use leftovers to make a soup

333 cal, 26g carb, 29g pro, 13g fat, 4g sat'd, .1g trans, 87mg chol, 4g fiber, 3g sugar, 380mg Na

CHICKEN FAJITAS

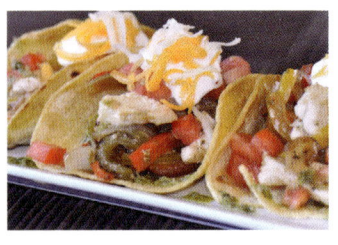

Prep time: 30 minutes
Makes 4 servings

1 Tbs	Seasoning, see page 47
¼ C	water
1 Lb	boneless skinless chicken breast, cut into strips
½	green bell pepper, strips
½	red bell pepper, strips
1	onion, sliced
1 Tbs	canola oil
2 Tbs	lime juice
4 Tbs	Green Salsa, see page 51
1 C	tomatoes, diced
4	whole-wheat tortillas
4 tsp	non-fat sour cream
½ C	low-fat shredded cheese

1. In a re-sealable bag, combine the seasoning and water. Add chicken, bell peppers, and onion to bag and gently knead to coat. Refrigerate for 15 minutes.
2. Heat oil in a skillet on high, add chicken and vegetables and cook. Cook until the vegetables are tender crisp and the chicken is cooked through.
3. Add lime juice, Green Salsa, and tomatoes, heat through.
4. Meanwhile, heat up a skillet and warm up tortillas.
5. Divide mixture evenly among tortillas. Top each with 1 Tsp sour cream and 2 Tbs shredded cheese. Roll up and serve.

260 cal, 35g carb, 14g pro, 9g fat, 2g sat'd, 0g trans, 22mg chol, 5g fiber, 5g sugar, 475mg Na

TURKEY CHILI

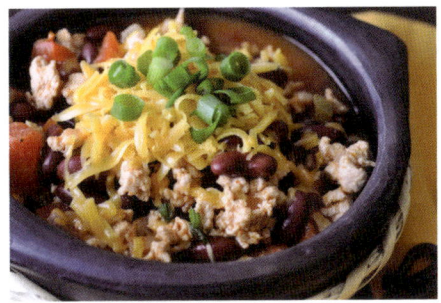

Prep time: 45 minutes
Makes 6 servings (serving size: 1 cup)

1 Tbs	canola oil
1 C	yellow onion, chopped
1 C	combination of bell peppers, chopped
½	stalk of celery, chopped
1 C	clove garlic
½ Lb	fat free ground turkey breast
14 ½ Oz	can diced tomato, no salt added
8 Oz	can tomato sauce, no salt added
15 ½ Oz	can kidney beans, rinsed and drained
2 C	water
2 Tbs	Seasoning, see page 47
½ C	low-fat shredded cheddar cheese
4 Tbs	fresh cilantro or green onion, chopped

1. Add oil to a large pot, and sauté onion, peppers, celery, and garlic over medium-high heat. Add turkey and cook until browned and vegetables are softened.
2. Stir in the tomatoes with their juice, tomato sauce, beans, water, and Seasoning. Bring to a boil. Cover, turn down the heat to medium-low, and cook for 20 minutes. Stirring occasionally.
3. Ladle into bowls, topping each serving with 2 Tbsp cheese and sprinkle with cilantro or green onion.

205 cal, 23g carb, 18g pro, 6g fat, 2g sat'd, 0g trans, 26mg chol, 7g fiber, 6g sugar, 294mg Na

TURKEY AND CORN QUESADILLAS

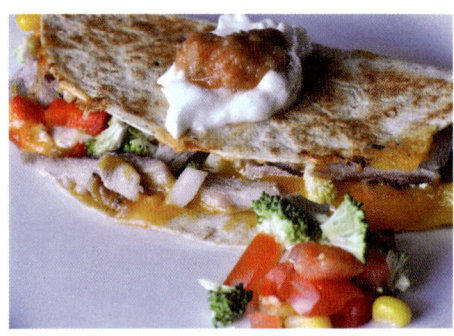

Prep time: 20 minutes
Makes 4 servings

4	whole-wheat tortillas
½ C	shredded reduced-fat cheddar cheese
1 C	shredded cooked 93% lean turkey breast
1 C	thawed frozen corn kernels
1 C	jarred roasted red pepper, chopped
4 Tbs	cilantro, chopped
¼ C	fat-free sour cream
½ C	Roasted Tomato Oregano Chunky Sauce, see page 50

1. Top half of each tortilla with ¼ C of cheddar cheese, ¼ C of turkey, ¼ of the corn, ¼ of the peppers, and 1 Tbs of the cilantro.
2. Fold the unfilled half over the filled half of tortilla, lightly pressing down.
3. Spray a large nonstick skillet with nonstick spray and set over medium heat. Add 2 quesadillas and cook until the tortillas are crisp and the cheese begins to melt, about 1-½ minutes on each side. Repeat with the remaining 2 quesadillas
4. Cut each quesadilla in half and transfer to a platter. Serve with sour cream and Roasted Tomato Oregano Chunky Sauce.

285 cal, 37g carb, 19g pro, 8g fat, 3g sat'd, .1g trans, 43mg chol, 5g fiber, 5g sugar, 375mg Na

Time Crunch?
Buy the rotisserie turkey breast.

TORTILLA CHIP-CRUSTED CHICKEN WITH GREEN SALSA

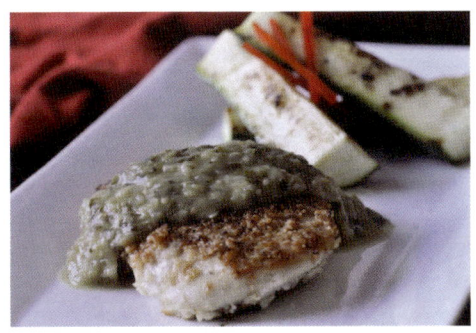

Prep time: 30 minutes
Makes 4 servings

4	Boneless chicken breasts, skinless, trimmed
1	egg white
2 Tbs	water or fat free milk
½ C	low-fat tortilla chips (2.5g fat), ground
3 tsp	canola oil
½ C	Green Salsa; see page 51

1. Place chicken between sheets of plastic wrap and pound with something heavy until flattened to an even thickness.
2. In a shallow dish whisk egg white and water until combined. Mix ground tortillas ships and salt in another dish. Dip each chicken breast in liquid, then dredge in ground tortilla, turning to coat evenly.
3. In a skillet, heat oil over medium heat. Cook chicken on both sides until browned on the outside and no longer pink in the middle. To get a moist chicken breast finish in an oven at 350 for 7 minutes, let rest and serve.
4. Serve the chicken with the Green Salsa, and any side you like.

235 cal, 9g carb, 27g pro, 10g fat, 1g sat'd, 0g trans, 76mg chol, 2g fiber, 1g sugar, 260mg Na

CHILAQUILES

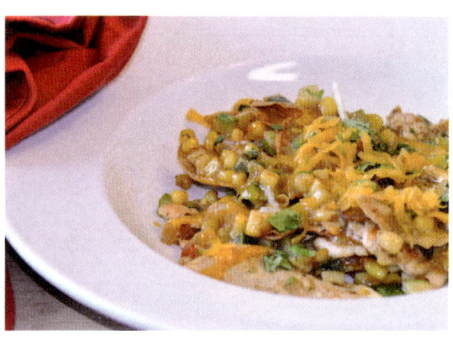

Prep time: 30 minutes
Makes 10 servings

2 tsp	Canola oil
1	yellow onion, chopped
1	zucchini, chopped
2 C	tomatoes, chopped
2 C	leftover chicken
1 ½ C	fresh corn
1 ½ tsp	Seasoning, see page 47
3	dozen corn tortillas, preferably left out overnight to dry out a bit, quartered or cut into 6 wedges
1 C	Green Salsa, see page 51
1 C	shredded reduced-fat cheddar cheese
	handful of cilantro

1. Heat oil in a large skillet over medium-high heat. Add onion and cook, until soft. Stir in zucchini, tomatoes with juice, chicken, corn and seasoning and cook, stirring occasionally, until the vegetables are cooked. Then add dried tortilla wedges, Green Salsa, and cheese. Stir until covered with the sauce; cover and let cook for about 5 minutes. They should be soft but not mushy.
2. Spoon some of the tortilla mixture onto a plate. Top with cilantro.

Saucy Suggestion:
Serve with greens and **Cilantro Dressing, see page 55,** and **Mango Salsa, see page 54.**

194 calories, 24g carb, 11g pro, 7g fat, 2g sat'd, 0 trans, 17mg chol, 4.3g fiber, 151mg Na

LIME ROASTED CHICKEN WITH GREEN SALSA

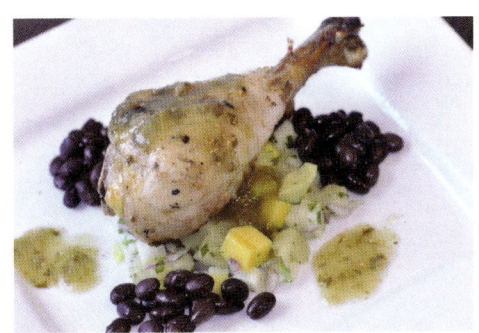

Prep time: 1 ½ hours
Makes 4 servings

4	*chicken legs, thighs, or breast with skin*
2 tsp	*canola oil*
1 Tbs	*lime zest*
2 tsp	**Seasoning, see page 47**
2	*garlic cloves, minced*
½ C	**Green Salsa, see page 51**
1	*serving* **Yellow Rice, see page 62**

1. Preheat oven to 375
2. Combine oil, Seasoning, lime zest, and garlic in a small bowl. Rub seasoning mixture under loosened skin. Place chicken, skin side up, on a pan with cooking spray. Bake for 40 minutes or until meat thermometer registers 165. Remove chicken from oven, let stand 10 minutes.
3. Remove and discard skin from chicken, and serve with Green Salsa on top, and Yellow Rice and black beans.

193 calories, 8 g carb, 18 g pro, 10 g, 2 g sat'd, 0 tans, 80 mg chol, 3 g fiber, 201 mg Na

BEEF

CHALUPAS

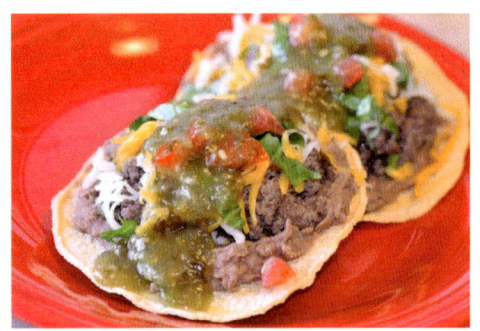

Prep time: 30 minutes
Makes 8 servings

1Lb	95 % lean ground beef
1 ¼ tsp	Seasoning, see page 47
8	corn tortillas
2C	Refried Beans, see page 49
½ C	shredded light Mexican cheese blend
2C	shredded romaine lettuce
2	tomatoes, diced
½	medium yellow onion, diced
¼ C	fresh cilantro, chopped
1	jalapeno, sliced
½ C	Green Salsa portion, see page 51

1. Brown ground beef in a large skillet, stirring to crumble. Sprinkle with the Seasoning and stir. Drain well, and set aside.
2. Warm refried beans in microwave or on stove top.
3. Place the tortillas on a cooking sheet and bake at 375 for 8 – 10 minutes.
4. Spread each tortilla with refried beans and ground beef. Top with cheese, lettuce, tomatoes, onions, cilantro, and jalapenos.
5. Serve with 1Tbs Green Salsa per serving.

288 cal, 28g carb, 24g pro, 9g fat, 4g sat'd, 2g trans, 48mg chol, 6g fiber, 3g sugar, 331mg Na

MEAT LOAF

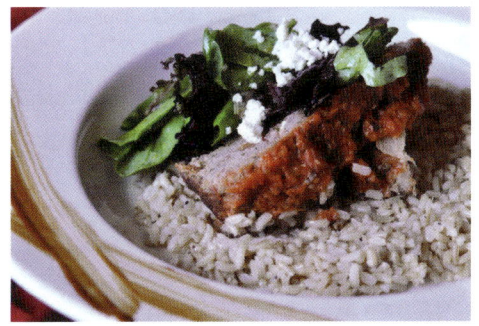

Prep time: 1 ½ hours
Makes 12 servings

1 ½ Lb 95% lean ground beef
1 ½ C   coarse breadcrumbs
½ C   yellow onion, chopped
1/3 C   parsley, chopped
1 Tbs   Dijon mustard
3   ripe tomatoes, chopped
3   medium chili peppers, seeded and chopped
tsp   salt
2   egg whites
½ C   **Roasted Tomato Oregano Chunky Sauce, (see page 50) pureed.**

Cooking spray

1. Preheat oven to 365
2. Combine beef, breadcrumbs, onions, parsley, Dijon mustard, tomatoes, peppers, salt, and egg whites in a bowl and hand mix.
3. Shape meat mixture into a loaf pan coated with cooking spray.
4. Bake 50 minutes, and then remove from oven; drain excess water and grease. Spoon **Roasted Tomato Oregano Chunky Sauce** over the meat loaf. Bake for 10 more minutes.
5. Before serving, let stand for 10 minutes, then cut loaf into 12 slices.

Saucy Suggestion:
☙ Serve with greens and **Cilantro Dressing, see page 55,** and **Brown Rice, see page 63**.

239 calories, 6 g carb, 34 g pro, 8 g fat, 3.4 g sat'd, .6 g trans, 92 mg chol, 1.4 g fiber, 270 mg Na

STUFFED PEPPERS WITH MANGO SALSA

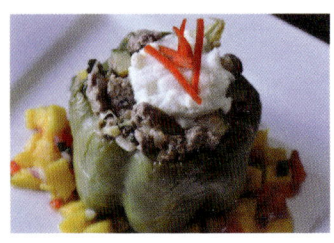

Prep time: 50 minutes
Makes 6 servings (serving size 1 cup)

2 Tbs	extra virgin olive oil
3	cloves garlic, minced
3	small zucchini, chopped
1 ½	medium yellow onion, chopped
1 can	quartered artichoke hearts, drained
2 ½ C	95 % lean ground beef
4 ½ C	Roasted Tomato Oregano Chunky Sauce, puree, see page 50
6 C	baby spinach
1 tsp	dried oregano
1 tsp	dijon mustard
½ C	fat-free ricotta cheese
6	bell peppers
1 ½ C	Mango Salsa, see page 54

1. Preheat oven to 350
2. Heat a saucepan over medium heat, add oil and garlic; cook until browns slightly. Add zucchini, artichokes, and onions; sauté until onions become translucent. Drain.
3. Add beef, stir, and cook until beef is browned. Mix in Roasted Tomato Chunky Oregano Sauce and baby spinach. Turn the heat to low and simmer for 10 minutes. Season with dried oregano and Dijon mustard.
4. Meanwhile, slice the tops off the peppers and remove core, seeds, and white membrane. Place peppers in a baking dish with ¼ inch of water in the pan. Fill each pepper with meat/vegetable sauce. Bake in the oven for 30 minutes. Spoon 1 Tbs of cheese onto each pepper, and then bake for another 10 minutes.
5. Serve peppers on top of the Mango Salsa.

333 calories, 35 g carb, 26 g pro, 12 g fat, 4 g sat'd, .1 g trans, 57 mg chol, 12 g fiber, 459 mg Na

CHORIZO MIGAS

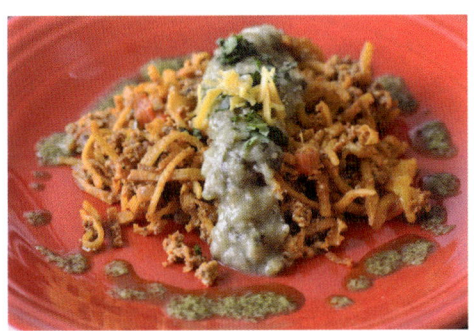

Prep time: 30 minutes
Makes 8 servings (serving size: 1 cup)

6	corn tortillas, cut into strips
1 Tbs	canola oil
½ Lb	leaner chorizo, casings removed
1	yellow onion, chopped
2	jalapeno, seeded, minced
2	tomatoes, chopped
8	eggs, beaten
½ tsp	dried oregano
½ tsp	salt
½ tsp	ground black pepper
1 C	low-fat cheddar cheese, shredded (optional)
½ C	cilantro, chopped
¼ C	Green Salsa per serving, see page 51

1. In a large skillet, heat oil and cook tortillas over medium heat, moving often, until lightly crispy. Drain on paper towels. Remove excess oil from skillet.
2. Cook chorizo in skillet on medium heat until lightly browned; drain. Add onion and jalapeno; cook for 2 minutes. Stir in tomatoes; cook for 2 minutes.
3. Add fried tortilla strips, eggs, oregano, salt, and pepper to skillet. Cook, stirring occasionally until eggs are almost set. Sprinkle with cheese; cover. Cook until cheese is melted.
4. Serve with **Green Salsa** and sprinkle with cilantro.

Saucy Suggestion:
Serve with the **Roasted Tomato Chunky Sauce, see page 50.**

252 calories, 15 g carb, 14 g pro, 15 g fat, 5 g sat'd, .4 g trans, 207 mg chol, 2.4 g fiber, 649 mg Na

LETTUCE WRAPS

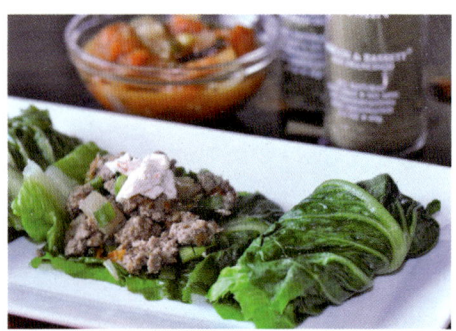

Prep time: 30 minutes
Serves 6 (serving size- 2 wraps)

2 Lb	95 % lean ground beef
2	onion, chopped
2	clove garlic, minced
2 tsp	Seasoning, see page 47
1	bunch green onion, chopped
4 C	Roasted tomato oregano chunky sauce, see page 50
12	lettuce leaves, washed and drained
½ C	goat cheese

1. In a large skillet, spray oil and brown ground beef, onion, green onion, and garlic. Drain well. Add Seasoning and the Roasted Tomato Oregano Chunky Sauce; mix well. Cook on low heat for 15 minutes to blend flavors.
2. Place one lettuce leaf on plate. Place meat mixture in center of leaf and add cheese. Roll up and serve.

Saucy Suggestion:
Serve leftovers over whole grain pasta and with shredded cheddar cheese.

381 calories, 30 g carb, 40 g pro, 8 g fat, 6 g sat'd, .5 g trans, 103 mg chol, 8 g fiber, 442 mg Na

PASTA WITH GROUND BEEF AND TOMATO SAUCE

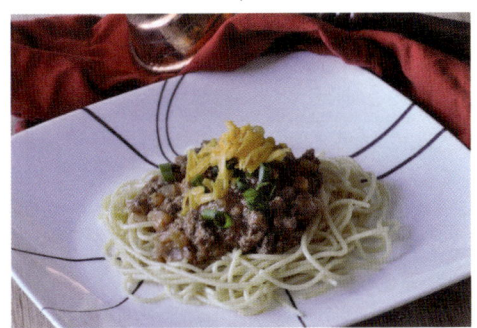

Prep time 30 minutes
4 servings

6 oz	95% lean ground beef
½	yellow onion, chopped
½	yellow bell pepper, chopped
2	garlic cloves, minced
1.5 C	**Roasted tomato oregano chunky sauce, see page 50**
2 tsp	**Seasoning, see page 47**
8 oz	spaghetti noodles
2 Tbs	green onion sliced
¼ C	shredded cheddar cheese 2%

1. In a saucepan, cook beef, onion, pepper, and garlic over medium heat until beef is browned. Drain off fat. Stir in Roasted Tomato Oregano Chunky Sauce and Seasoning. Bring to boil; reduce heat. Simmer until desired consistency, stirring occasionally.
2. Meanwhile, cook pasta in boiling salted water. Drain.
3. Serve pasta on the plate topped with sauce, sprinkle green onions and cheese.

349 calories, 58 g carb, 22 g pro, 5 g fat, 2 g sat'd, .2 g trans, 30 mg chol, 4 g fiber, 269 mg Na

FISH

GRILLED FISH TACOS

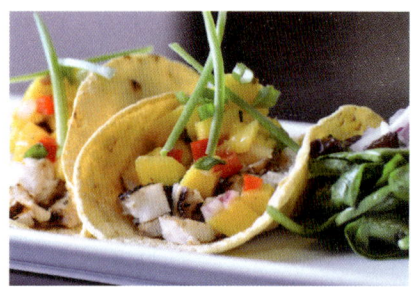

Prep time: 40 minutes
Serves 6

¼ C	canola oil
1.5 tsp	**Seasoning, see page 47**
1 Tbs	lemon juice
1	jalapeno, chopped
¼ C	fresh cilantro, chopped
1 Lb	red snapper, 2-inch wide strips
12	corn tortillas, warmed
1.5 C	cabbage, shredded

1. Preheat grill to medium-high.
2. Place fish in a medium size dish; set aside. In a small bowl whisk together oil, **Seasoning**, lemon juice, jalapeno, and cilantro and pour over the fish. And let marinate for 10 minutes. Drain fish, discarding any marinade. Grill the fish until it is just cooked through (approx. 4 minutes per side) or until fish flakes easily with a fork. Let rest for 5 minutes; flake fish with a fork.

Saucy Suggestion:
- Serve in warmed tortillas topped with Jicama Pineapple, **Mango Salsa, see page 47, Guacamole, see page 48, and Coleslaw, see page 52.**
- You can use flounder, tilapia, halibut or mahi-mahi instead of red-snapper.

192 cal, 23g carb, 19g pro, 3g fat, .5g sat'd, 0g trans, 28mg chol, 4g fiber, 1g sugar, 83mg Na

RECIPES

RED SNAPPER VERACRUZ-STYLE

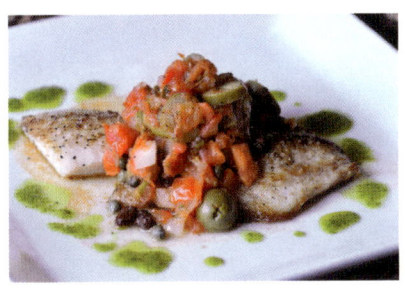

Prep time: 30 minutes
Serves 4

½ C	tomato puree (from fresh tomatoes)
4	ripe tomatoes, diced
4 tsp	extra-virgin olive oil
4	4 oz red snapper fillets
1 tsp	salt
1	small white onion, thinly sliced
3	garlic cloves, chopped
4	bay leaves
1 tsp	dried oregano
¼ C	pitted green olives, chopped
2 Tbs	raisins
2 Tbs	drained capers
2 Tbs	fresh cilantro, chopped

1. Preheat the oven to 425
2. Season fish with salt.
3. First place the tomatoes in a blender and puree, add water if needed to give a pureed consistency.
4. In a skillet, heat the oil over medium-high heat, add the snapper and sear both sides until golden brown, then remove and keep warm.
5. In the same skillet, add onion and stir 30 seconds. Add garlic and stir 30 seconds. Add tomato puree and cook 1 minute. Add bay leaves, oregano, and diced tomatoes. Simmer until sauce thickens. Add olives, raisins, and capers. Simmer until sauce thickens again, stirring occasionally. Season to taste with salt and black pepper.
6. Spread some sauce in bottom of glass baking dish. Arrange fish on top of sauce. Spoon remaining sauce over. Cover with aluminum foil and bake until fish cooks, about 15 minutes
7. Transfer fish with sauce to plates and sprinkle with cilantro.

Saucy Suggestion:
- The sauce is also great with grilled chicken or grilled fish.
- **Brown rice is a good side for this fish. See page 63.**

222 cal, 14g carb, 26g pro, 8g fat, 1g sat'd, 0g trans, 42mg chol, 3g fiber, 8g sugar, 928mg Na

PORK

PORK CHOPS WITH CORN-BELL PEPPER RELISH

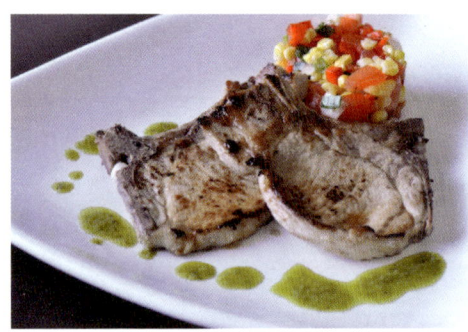

Prep time: 35 minutes
Serves 4

2 Tbs	extra-virgin olive oil
1 T	orange juice
2 Tbs	sherry vinegar
2 tsp	garlic, chopped
½ tsp	Seasoning, see page 47
2 C	Corn Bell Pepper Relish, see page 53
4	thin-cut boneless pork loin chops, trimmed

1. Combine oil, orange juice, vinegar, garlic, and Seasoning in a blender; process until creamy. Rub both sides of pork chops with sauce. Marinate for 10 minutes. Drain.
2. Spray oil in a large nonstick skillet over medium-high heat. Add the pork chops and cook until browned and cook through, about 3 minutes on each side.
3. Serve with Corn Bell Pepper Relish.

299 cal, 16g carb, 21g pro, 17g fat, 3g sat'd, 0g trans, 48mg chol, 2g fiber, 6g sugar, 122 mg Na

VEGETARIAN

REFRIED BEAN AND BUTTERNUT TACOS

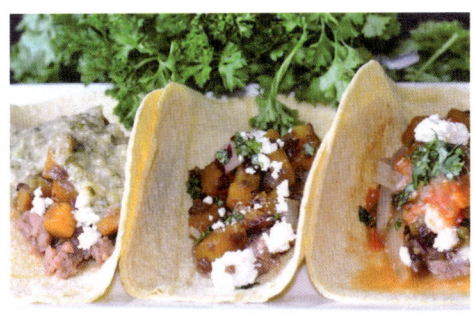

Prep time: 30 minutes
Serves 8

1 Tbs	extra virgin olive oil
½ C	red onion, chopped
2	garlic cloves, chopped
2 C	small butternut squash, peeled, seeded, cut into ½" cubes
1 ½ tsp	coriander
½ tsp	cinnamon
2 tsp	Seasoning, see page 47
1 ½ C	Refried Beans, see page 49
8	corn tortillas
½ C	cilantro leaves
¾ C	feta cheese

1. Add the oil to a skillet, and sauté the red onion and garlic until browned. Then add the squash and sauté until cooked through, stirring frequently. Mix in coriander, cinnamon, and Seasoning.
2. While the squash is cooking, heat up the refried beans in a saucepan or in the microwave.
3. Warm the tortillas one at a time in a skillet over medium heat. Keep warm.
4. Spoon some of the beans into each tortilla. add the squash and sprinkle some cilantro and cheese.

Saucy Suggestion:
- Replace Refried Beans with rinsed, canned Black Beans.
- You can serve with **Roasted Tomato Oregano Chunky Sauce, see page 50**, and/or **Green Salsa, see page 51.**
- For lunch serve one taco with **Yellow Rice, see page 62** and **Coleslaw, see page 52.**

> ⏲ **Time Crunch?**
> Buy Frozen Chopped Butternut Squash

183 cal, 27g carb, 7 g pro, 6g fat, 3g sat'd, 0g trans, 0mg chol, 5g fiber, 3g sugar, 252mg Na

VEGETABLE QUESADILLA

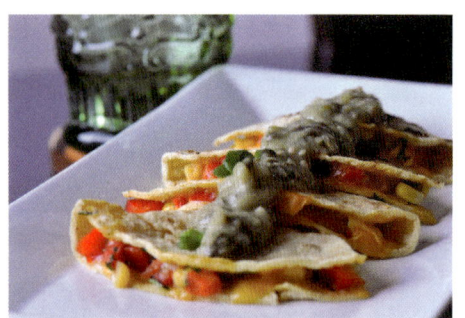

Prep time: 20 minutes
Serves 6

2	*tomatoes, seeded, diced*
½ C	*red onion, chopped*
½ C	*roasted red peppers, sliced*
1	*head of broccoli, chopped*
½ C	*kernel corn frozen*
½ C	*zucchini, sliced*
6	*corn tortillas*
12	*Tbs reduced fat jack cheese shredded for each quesadilla*

1. Preheat oven at 400.
2. Mix red bell peppers with little oil and roast for 10 minutes. Meanwhile on a skillet with oil spray, quickly sauté the vegetables until tender. Season with dash of salt.
3. Coat a large skillet with cooking spray. Set pan over medium heat to preheat. Add the tortillas and warm up, then top each tortilla with an equal amount of vegetables and 2 Tbs cheese. Fold over tortillas. Cook until golden brown each side and cheese melts.

244 cal, 33g carb, 14g pro, 7g fat, 4g sat'd, 0g trans, 18mg chol, 5g fiber, 4g sugar, 351mg Na

REFRIED BEAN BURGERS WITH GUACAMOLE

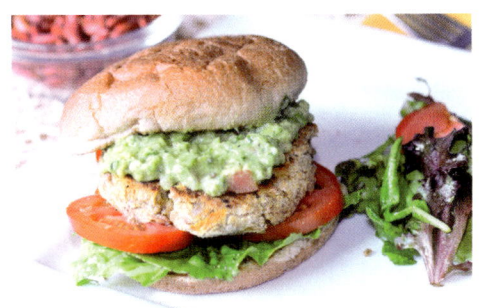

Prep time: 40 minutes
Serves 6

1	*large red onion, finely chopped*
1 Tbs	*canola oil*
2	*garlic cloves, minced*
1	*medium carrot, shredded*
2 tsp	Seasoning, see page 47
2 ½ C	Refried Beans, see page 49
2 Tbs	*Dijon mustard*
3 Tbs	*cilantro, chopped*
3 Tbs	*cornmeal, ⅓ C for coating burgers*
½	*tsp salt*
6	*whole-wheat hamburger buns, toasted*
6	*lettuce leaves*
6	*tomatoes slices*
1 ¼ C	Guacamole, see page 48

1. In a large skillet sauté onion in oil, for 2 minutes. Add garlic; cook for 1-minute stir in the carrot, and Seasoning; cook until carrot is tender. Remove from heat; set aside.
2. In a large bowl, add the refried beans, mustard, cilantro, cornmeal, and carrot mixture; mix well. Shape into 6 patties. Coat them evenly with the remaining 1/3 C cornmeal.
3. In a skillet coated with spray over medium-high heat, cook burgers until brown and crisp on both sides, 2 to 4 minutes per side.
4. Serve the burgers on buns with lettuce, tomatoes and Guacamole.

408 calories, 67 g carb, 15 g pro, 11 g fat, 1.5 g sat'd, 0 trans, 0 chol, 14 g fiber, 680 mg Na,

Tortilla Trimmer:
Purchase 100 calorie buns to serve burger on to save some calories.

REFRIED BEAN CAKES WITH GUACAMOLE DRESSING

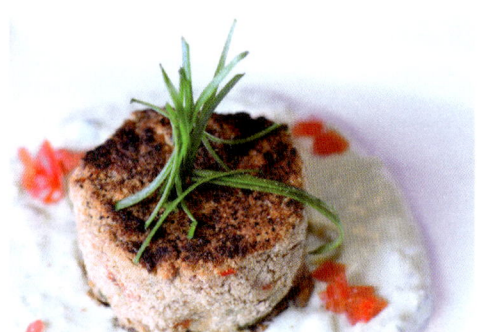

Prep time: 30 minutes
Serves 4

1 C	Guacamole, see page 48
¼ C	light sour cream
1 tsp	lime juice
2	slices whole wheat bread, crumbs
2 C	Refried beans, drained, see page 49
½	yellow onion, chopped
½	green bell pepper, diced
½	red bell pepper, diced
2	cloves garlic, minced
1.5 Tbs	vegetable oil
1.5 tsp	cumin
1	egg
1	tomato, diced
salt and pepper to taste	

1. Preheat the oven to 400.
2. Mix ¾ C of the Guacamole, sour cream, and lime juice. Set aside.
3. Sauté onions, peppers, and garlic in oil until tender over medium-high, and set aside to cool down.
4. Add the beans to the sautéed vegetables and mix in the breadcrumbs, cumin, salt and pepper, and mix well. Shape into four ½ inch thick patties.
5. In a skillet, with spray oil and sear patties for 1 minute on each side. The patties should have a golden brown crust. Place into the oven for about 5 minutes.
6. To serve, place the guacamole mixture on the plate, add the cake, and top off with a dab of guacamole with some diced tomatoes.

356 calories, 44 g carb, 14 g pro, 15 g fat, 3 g sat'd, .2 g trans, 46 mg chol, 11 g fiber, 329 mg Na

CHAPTER 9
LET'S BURN THOSE TORTILLAS!

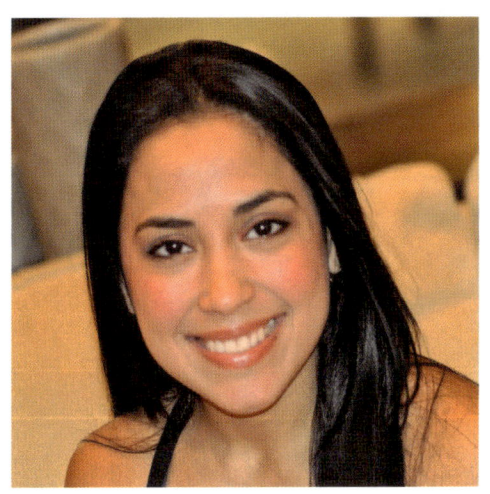

Lauren Flores is a Certified Personal Trainer and Group Fitness Instructor from Brownsville, Texas. She has 7 years of working in the fitness industry under her belt and has successfully helped numerous people lose weight by living a healthier lifestyle. She has further enhanced her life-goal of helping others and currently works as a Nutrition Coach at My Fit Foods in San Antonio, Texas. She enjoys being active, cooking and spending time her family. Lauren believes that to impact your overall health, your diet is 80% and your physical activity is 20%. Her motto is, "You are what you eat!"

How to use the fitness section of the book

We have created an easy to follow exercise program to get you through four weeks. Each week we have built two circuits (one upper body and one lower body). Do each circuit at least one time per week or two times a week, if possible. The circuits are built to give you strength training and cardio; however, if you can supplement with 30-45 minutes of cardio each week, you will see better results.

If you have a busy week and you have to decide between doing the circuits or cardio, always choose the circuits because when you build muscle, you increase your metabolism, and, therefore, burn more calories throughout the day. You will also see faster results because you are sculpting your body.

Once you have gone through the month of circuit training, you can either repeat the circuits using more repetitions or heavier weights, or you can look up ways to vary each of the exercises.

EQUIPMENT : Pair of dumbbells (3-15lbs) and chair (optional: exercise mat).

WORKOUT INSTRUCTIONS:

- Warm-up with a **10-15 minute walk or jog** and then hold a **plank for 1 minute** (modify the plank if you are a beginner, have a weak core, or have a bad back by leaving your knees on the ground)

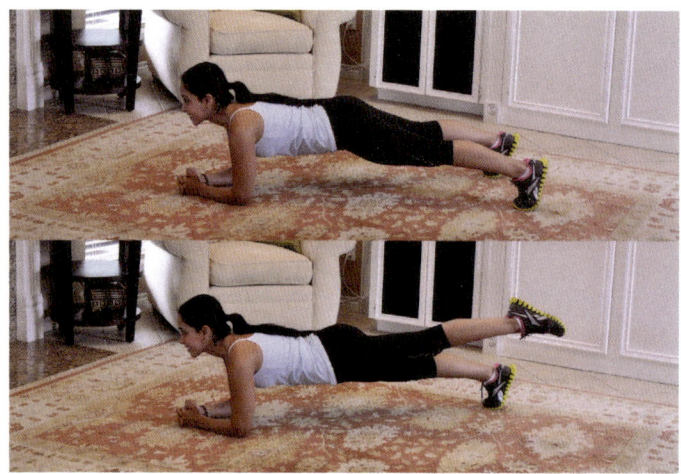

- Repeat each circuit **3-5 times** with a 30 second break in between each circuit.
- Aim for **12-15 repetitions** unless otherwise indicated.
- Cool down with a 10-minute walk or jog and stretch.
- Enjoy your workout!

WEEK 1

Circuit 1 (Upper Body)

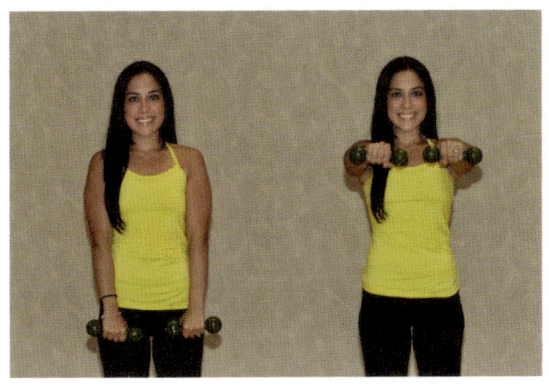

- SHOULDER FRONT RAISE: Starting position; feet hip width apart, slight bend in the knees, dumbbells at your thighs. Ending position; raise arms to shoulder level and release.

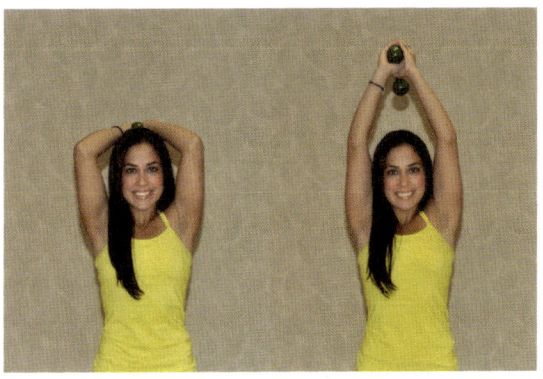

- OVERHEAD TRICEP EXTENSIONS: Starting position; dumbbell behind head, elbows pointing forward. Ending position; straighten arms and release.

HEALTHY TEX-MEX

- CARDIO: Jumping Jacks (30-45 seconds)

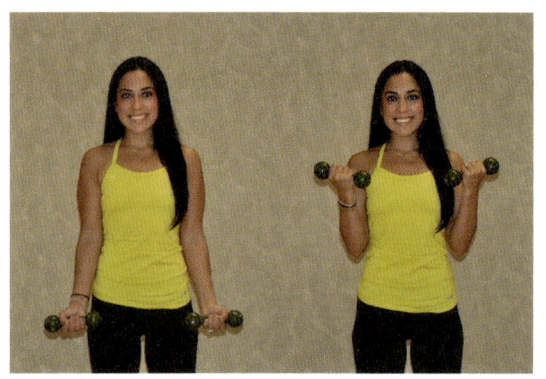

- DOUBLE BICEP CURLS: Starting position; feet hip width apart, slight bend in the knees, dumbbells at your thighs. Ending position; curl arms, dumbbells three inches from chest and release.

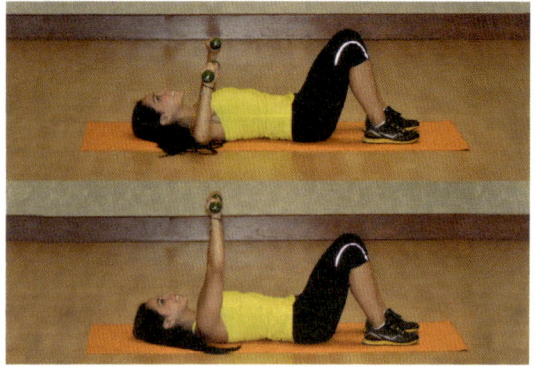

- CHEST PRESS: Starting position; on your back with your feet close to your bottom, arms in a 90 degree. Ending position; extend arms over body then release back to 90 degree position.

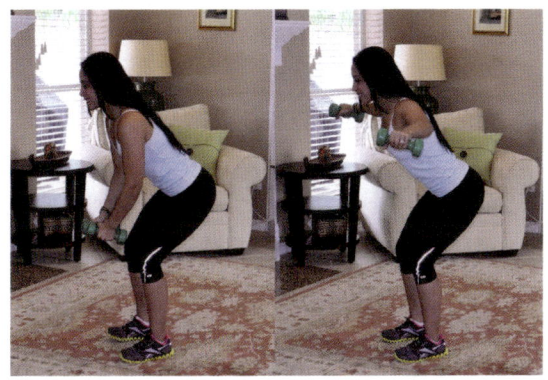

- BENT-OVER FLY: Starting position; feet hip width apart, slight bend in the knees, arms to the front with a slight bend in the arms, lean forward (back should be at 45 degree). Ending position; extend arms to your side, dumbbells up to shoulder height and release.

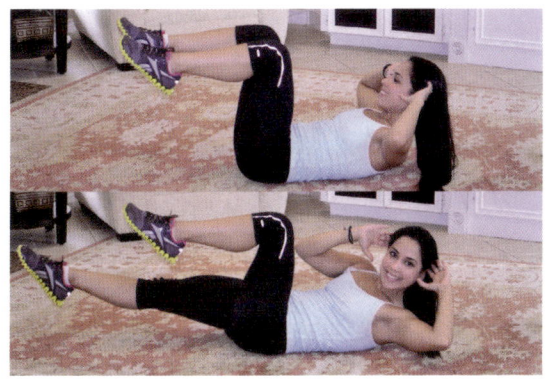

- BICYCLE CRUNCH: Starting position; legs up in a 90 degree with your fingertips to temple. Ending position; extend one leg and take to opposite elbow to the knee that is still bent then alternate. (Option: feet on ground lift one knee up and take opposite elbow to it then alternate).

- CARDIO: Jumping Jacks (30-45 seconds)

Circuit 2 (Lower Body)

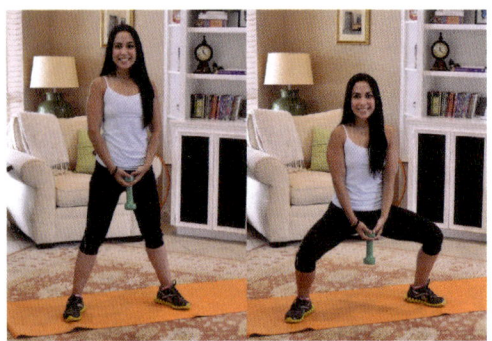

- DUMBBELL SUMO SQUATS: Starting position; feet slightly wider than hips, toes slightly pointed out, arms to front with dumbbells in hand. Ending position; lower bottom to about chair height then release, pull up with your heels and squeeze gluteus maximus as you rise. (Option: since we're working a big muscle group, use one dumbbell if you want to up your weight rather than using two 10 pound dumbbells).

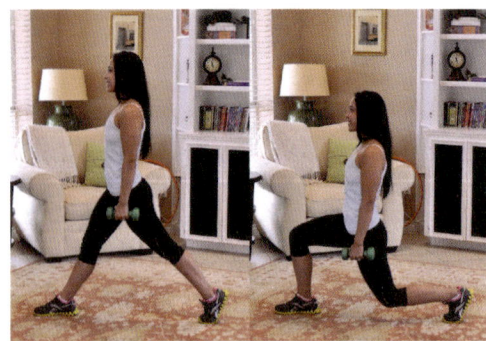

- LUNGES WITH DUMBBELL: Starting position; one leg to the front, the other to the back both slightly bent, arms out in a running position, lower body, front leg in a 90 degree (knee above foot) back leg still slightly bent. Ending position; bring back knee to the front of your body (90 degree) then release. (Option: toe tap floor)

- CARDIO: Jump rope (30-45 seconds) If you do not have a jump rope, just move your hands like you would with a rope during the exercise.

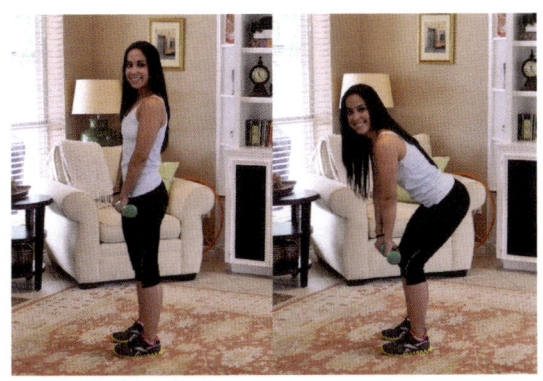

- DEADLIFT: Starting position; feet under shoulders and hip width apart, slight bend in the knees, dumbbells at your thighs. Ending position; lower upper body taking dumbbells right past the middle of your knees and release. (Option: since we're working a big muscle group, use heavier dumbbells if you'd like).

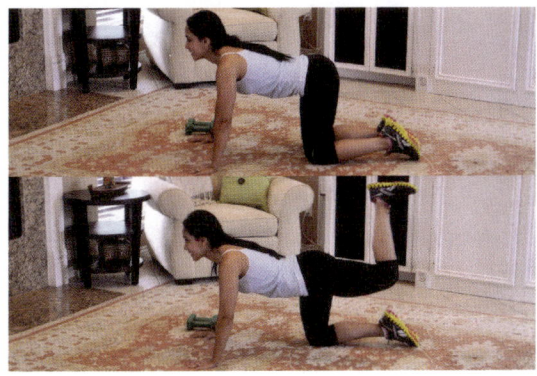

- GLUTE KICKBACK: Starting position; knees on floor. Lower chest to floor as if you're going into a pushup position (hands shoulder width apart). Bring knees to a 90-degree angle. Lift up your right leg until the hamstrings are in line with the back while maintaining the 90-degree angle bend. Contract the glutes throughout this movement and hold the contraction at the top for a second and release.

HEALTHY TEX-MEX

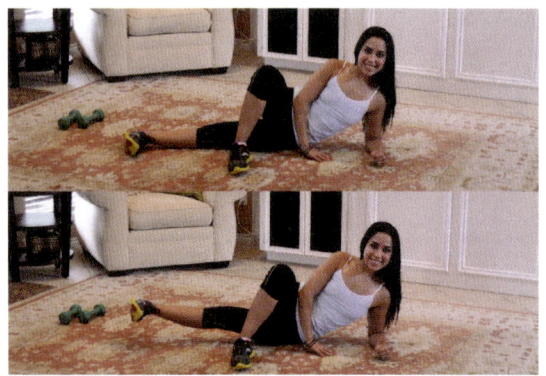

- ADDUCTOR LEG LIFT : Starting position; lay on one side with hand closest to floor to head and other hand resting on floor in front of torso. Keep bottom leg extended and bring the foot of your top leg as close as you can to the knee of the extended leg. Pulse extended leg 12-15 times and switch to other side.

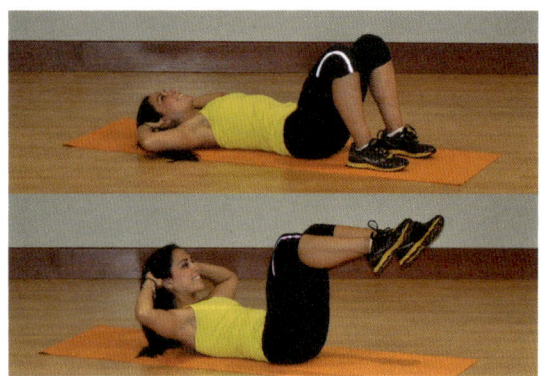

- C-CRUNCH: Starting position; feet on ground keep them close to your bottom with your fingertips to temple. Ending position; legs come up to a 90 degree as you crunch then release. (Option: keep feet on ground and crunch).

- CARDIO: Jump rope (30-45 seconds)

WEEK 2

Circuit 1 (Upper Body)

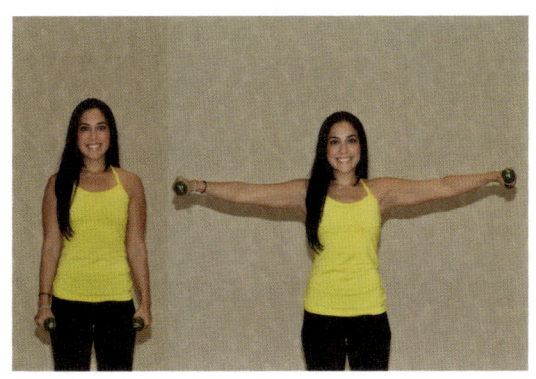

- **SHOULDER SIDE RAISE:** Starting position; feet under shoulders and hip width apart, slight bend in the knees, dumbbells on the side of your thighs. Ending position; raise arms to your side with a slight bend in the elbow and release.

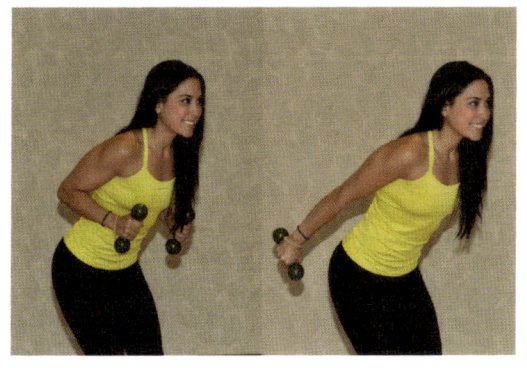

- **BENT-OVER TRICEP EXTENSION:** Starting position; feet under shoulders and hip width apart, slight bend in the knees, arms to your side in a 90 degree, lean forward (back should be at 45 degree). Ending position; extend both arms to back and release.

HEALTHY TEX-MEX

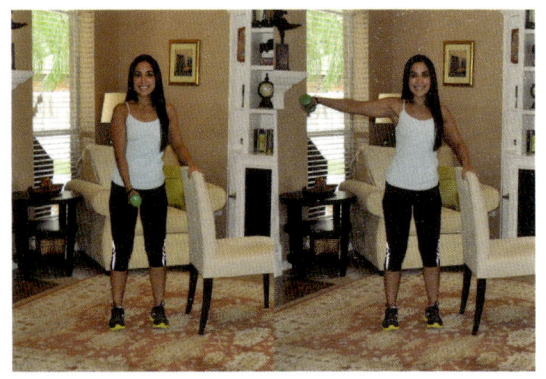

- SINGLE ARM HAMMER CURLS: Starting position; feet under shoulders and hip width apart, slight bend in the knees, dumbbells on the side of your thighs with the end of dumbbell facing the front of the room. Ending position; curl one arm and release then alternate to other arm.

- CARDIO: Jump squats (10-12 reps): Stand with your feet shoulder-width apart, arms resting on your hips. Start by doing a regular squat, then engage your core and jump up explosively. When you land, lower your body back into the squat position to complete one rep.

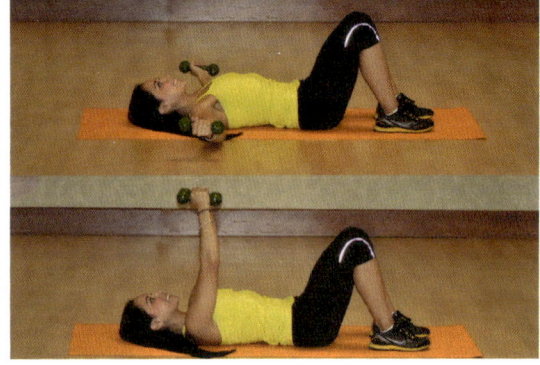

- CHEST FLY: Starting position; on your back with feet close to bottom, arms out to side (slight bend in elbows). Ending position; extend arms above body (dumbbells meet in center) and release.

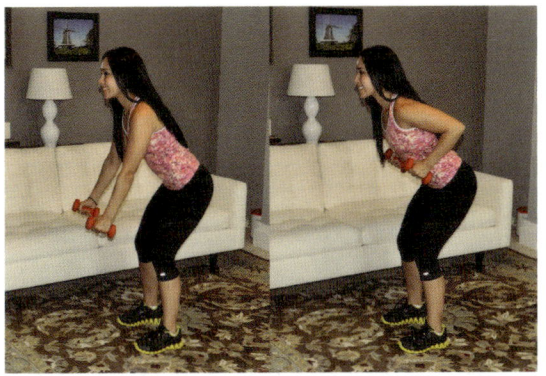

- BENT-OVER BACK ROW (neutral grip): Starting position; feet under shoulders and hip width apart, slight bend in the knees, arms to your side, lean forward (back should be at 45 degree). Ending position; bring dumbbells to side of ribs, keep elbows in, squeeze shoulder blades then release.

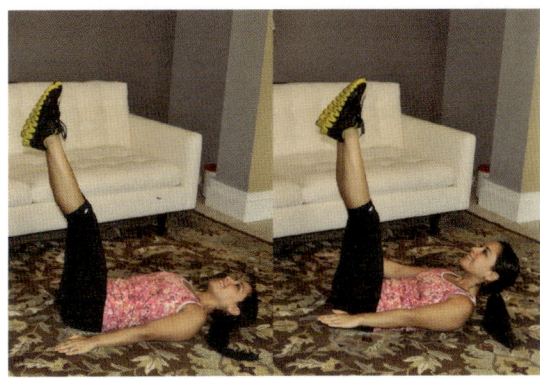

- VERTICAL LEG CRUNCH: Starting position; laying on back with feet 90 degrees in the air. Ending positing, using your abdominal muscle, slightly tilt your pelvis straight up.

- CARDIO: Jump squats (10-12 reps)

Circuit 2 (Lower Body)

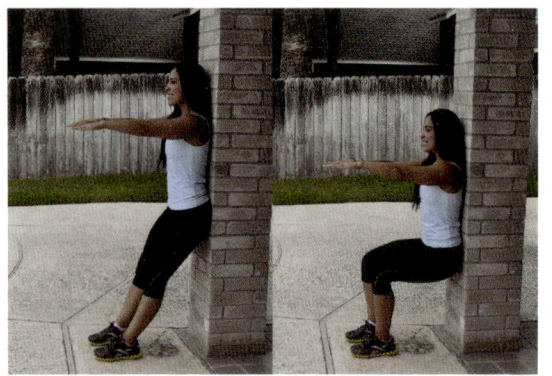

- WALL SQUATS (option: with dumbbells. Hold for 45 seconds): Sit against the wall with your legs at 90 degrees, as if you are sitting on a chair, and hold this position.

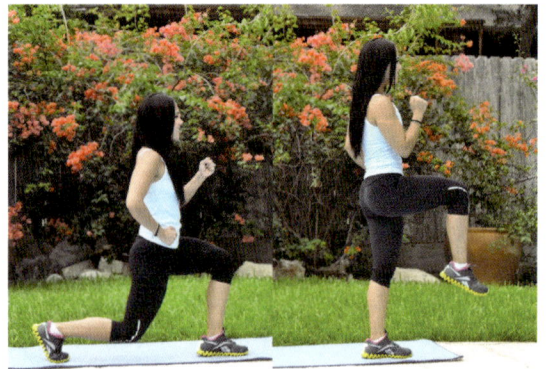

- DYNAMIC LUNGES: One leg to the front other to the back both slightly bent, arms out in a running position, lower body, front leg in a 90 degree (knee above foot) back leg still slightly bent. Ending position; bring back knee to the front of your body (90 degree) then release. (Option: toe tap floor)

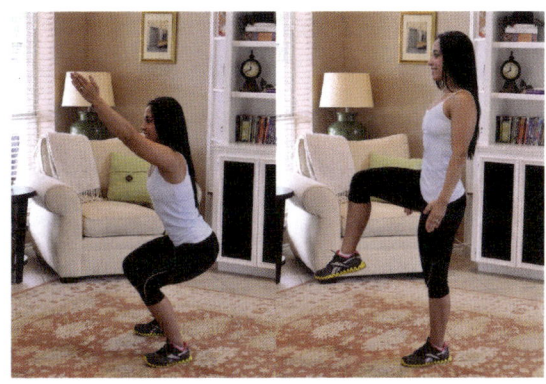

- **STANDING LEG LIFTS:** Starting position; feet hip width apart with hands on waist. Extend one leg to the back 45-degree angle with foot flexed. Ending position; hold and squeeze glutes and release.

- **CARDIO:** Jumping Lunges (10-15 reps) Stand with your feet together, elbows bent 90 degrees. Lunge forward with your right foot [A]. Jump straight up as you thrust your arms forward, elbows still bent. Switch legs in midair, like a scissor [B], and land in a lunge with your left leg forward [C]. Repeat, switching legs again. That's 1 rep. To prevent injury, try to land as softly as possible.

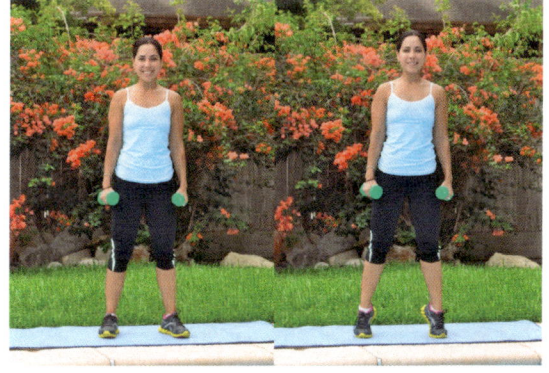

- **CALF RAISES WITH DUMBBELLS:** Starting position; feet hip width apart with toes slightly turned out. Ending position; lift heels off ground and release.

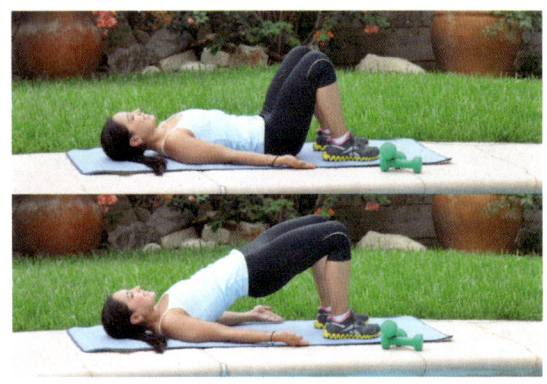

- BRIDGE: Starting position; Back on floor with feet in (close to the bottom). Arms on floor extended to your side. Ending position; lift your back and bottom off floor. Hold for 45 seconds and squeeze glutes.

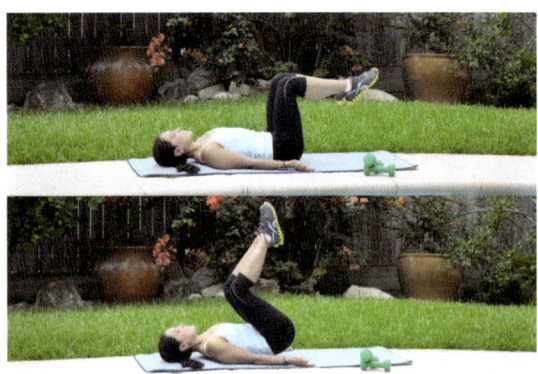

- REVERSE CURL: Starting position; Back on floor with legs up in a 90-degree angle. Arms on floor extended to your side. Ending position; lift your bottom off floor and bring your knees in toward your chest and release.

- CARDIO: Jumping Lunges (10-15 reps)

WEEK 3

Circuit 1 (Upper Body)

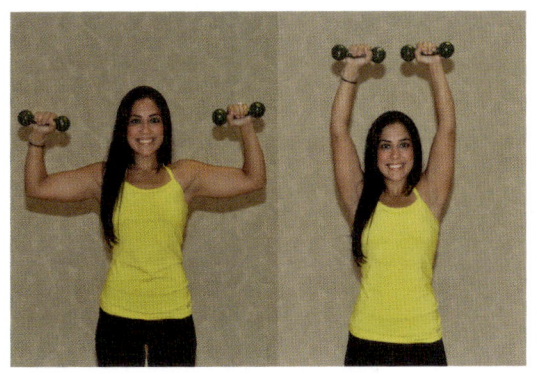

- SHOULDER PRESS: Starting position; feet under shoulders and hip width apart, slight bend in the knees, arms raised in a 90 degree position. Ending position; extend arms, meet dumbbells above your head and release to 90 degree position.

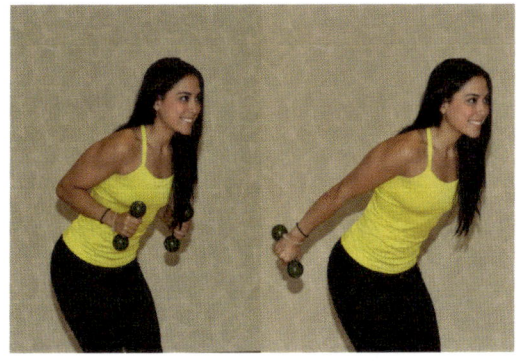

- TRICEP EXTENSIONS: Starting position; dumbbell behind head, elbows pointing forward. Ending position; straighten arms and release.

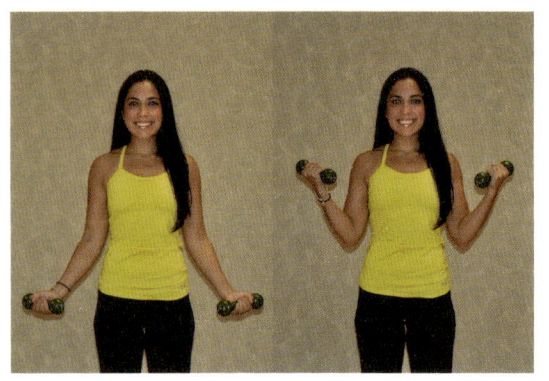

- LATERAL BICEP CURL: Starting position; feet under shoulders and hip width apart, slight bend in the knees, arms to your side, and elbows to ribs. Ending position; curl arms and release.

- CARDIO: Jump squats (10-12 reps): Stand with your feet shoulder-width apart, arms resting on your hips. Start by doing a regular squat, then engage your core and jump up explosively. When you land, lower your body back into the squat position to complete one rep.

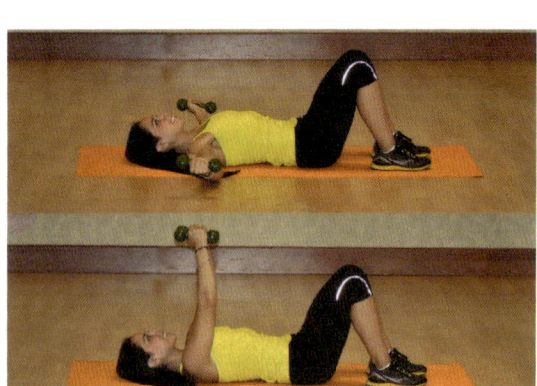

- CHEST FLY: Starting position; on your back with feet close to bottom, arms out to side (slight bend in elbows). Ending position; extend arms above body (dumbbells meet in center) and release.

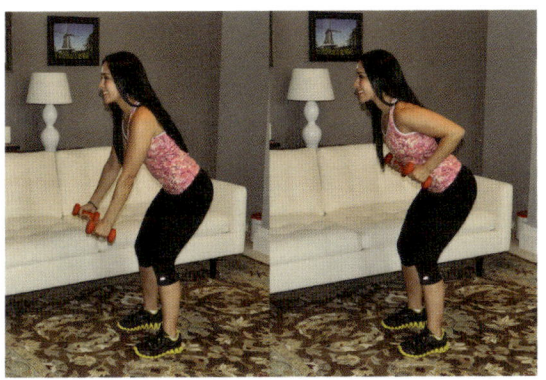

- BENT-OVER BACK ROW (reverse grip): Starting position; feet under shoulders and hip width apart, slight bend in the knees, arms to your side, lean forward (back should be at 45 degree). Ending position; bring dumbbells to side of ribs, keep elbows in, squeeze shoulder blades then release.

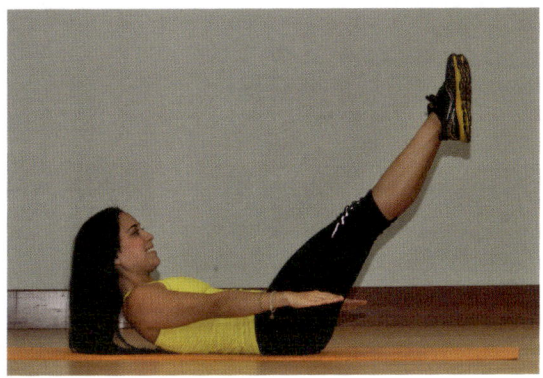

- PILATES 100'S: Starting position; Back on floor with legs extended in a 45-degree (option: legs vertical with toes to ceiling). Arms extended to side with hands off floor. Ending position; lift chest and shoulder blades off floor and pulse hands up and down.

- CARDIO: Jump squats (10-12 reps)

Circuit 2 (Lower Body)

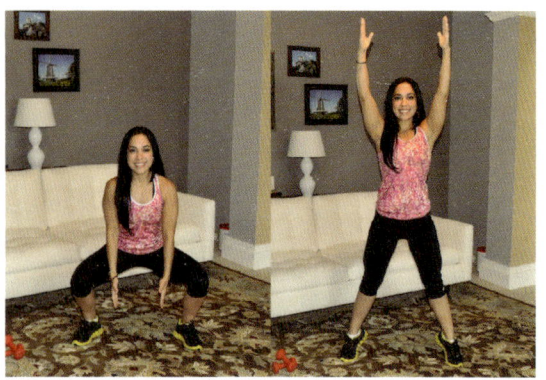

- GRAND PLIE SQUAT WITH REACH: Starting position; Feet wider than hips with toes slightly turned out. Lower your upper body and reach your arms between your legs. Ending position; Lift your upper body up, extend arms overhead and pull up to toes.

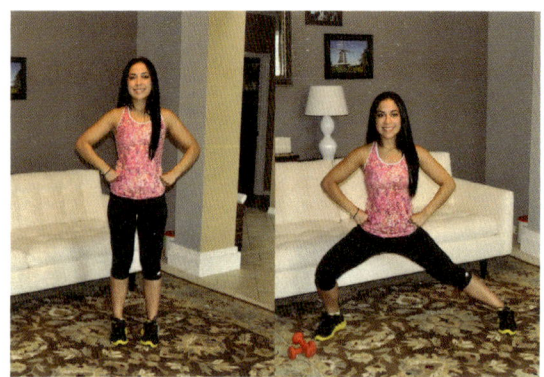

- ALTERNATING SIDE LUNGES: Starting position; feet under hips, step one foot to your side (bend knee to a 90-degree). Other leg is extended with foot on floor. Release to starting position and switch to other leg. (Option: dumbbells in hands)

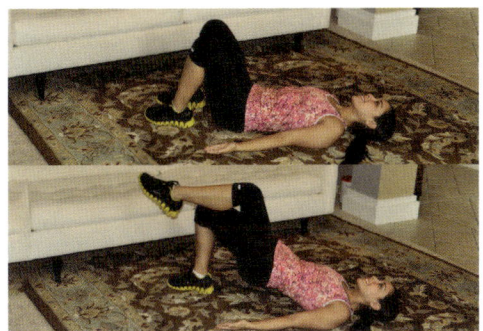

- **SINGLE KNEE BRIDGE WITH PULSE:** Starting position; Back on floor with feet in (close to the bottom). Arms on floor extended to your side. Ending position; lift your back and bottom off floor. At the same time you should have one leg elevated at 90-degree. Pulse 12-15 times. Release and repeat on other side.

- **CARDIO:** High knees (30-45 seconds): Stand tall with your feet shoulder-width apart. Without changing your posture, raise your left knee as high as you can and step forward. Repeat with your right leg. Continue to alternate back and forth. For more of a challenge, make each step a jump.

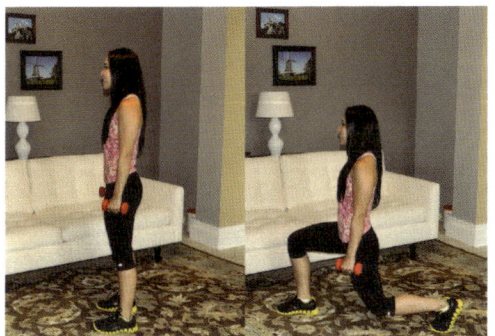

- **WALKING LUNGES WITH DUMBBELLS:** Starting position; one dumbbell in each hand and stand upright. Step forward with one foot. The toes of both feet should be facing straight ahead. Be sure your legs are aligned - your front knee should be aligned with the foot. Ending position; lower your back knee towards the floor. Push back up to the starting position and squeeze glutes then switch. As you switch you should be stepping forward as if you're walking.

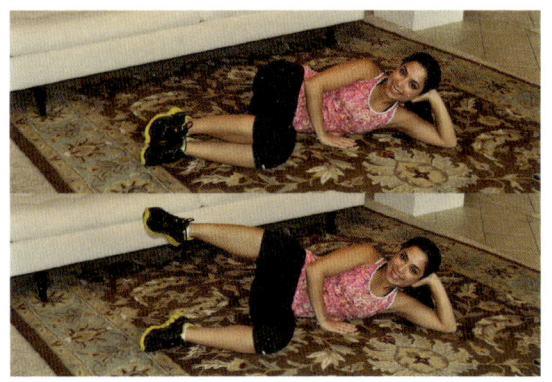

- **LEG CLAMS:** Starting position; Lay on side and bring legs to a 90-degree angle. Hand closest to floor should rest under head and other hand should rest on floor in front of torso. Ending position; lift top leg up and release.

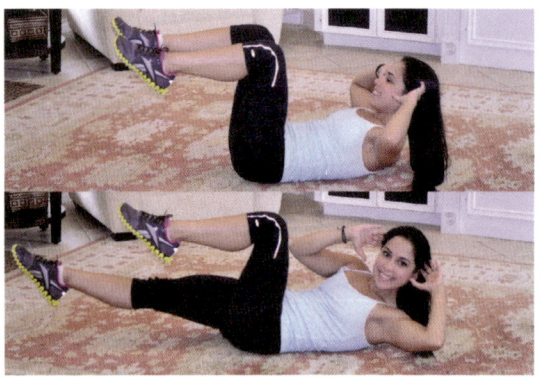

- **SIDE OBLIQUE CRUNCH:** Starting position; Lay on side and bring legs to a 90-degree angle. Extend bottom arm to front and back to head. Ending position; crunch to your side. Almost as if you're bringing your elbow to hip and release. Switch to other side.

- **CARDIO:** High knees (30-45 seconds)

WEEK 4

Circuit 1 (Upper Body)

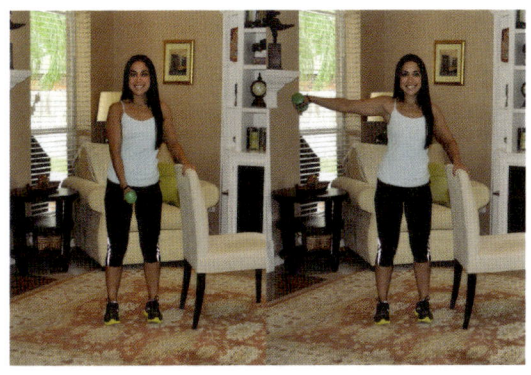

- SINGLE ARM DELTOID RAISE WITH CHAIR: Starting position; Feet slightly wider than hips. Place on hand on chair for balance and other hand (with dumbbell) in front of body. Ending position; Extend arm out to side and release then switch.

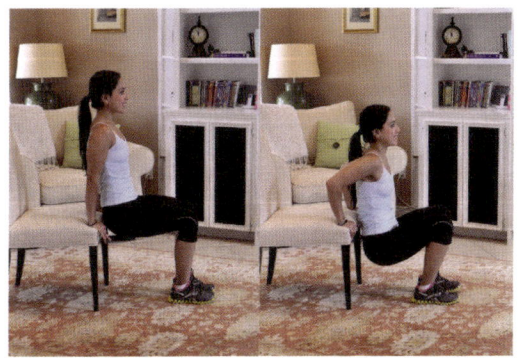

- TRICEP DIP WITH CHAIR: Starting position; Sit on edge of chair with hands to your side on chair. Ending position; pull your bottom off chair and dip until elbows are at 90-degree then release. (Option: dumbbell on lap)

HEALTHY TEX-MEX

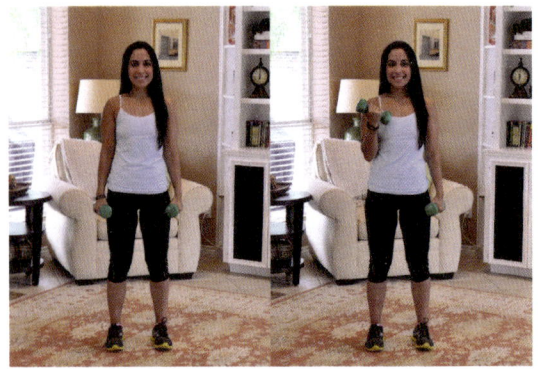

- SINGLE DUMBBELL BICEP CURL: Starting position; feet under shoulders and hip width apart, slight bend in the knees, dumbbells at your thighs. Ending position; curl arms, dumbbells three inches from chest and release.

- CARDIO: Mountain climbers (30-45 seconds): Place hands on floor, slightly wider than shoulder width. On forefeet, position one leg forward bent under body and extend other leg back. While holding upper body in place, alternate leg positions by pushing hips up while immediately extending forward leg back and pulling rear leg forward under body, landing on both forefeet simultaneously.

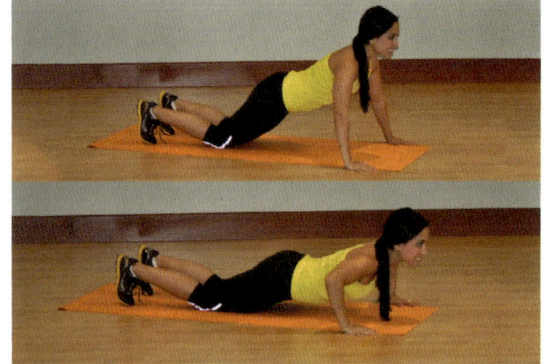

- PUSHUP: Starting position; plank position (hands under shoulders and feet hip width apart) with elbows pointing to the side of the room. Ending position; lower your body to floor and push back up. (Option: on knees feet on ground)

LET'S BURN THOSE TORTILLAS!

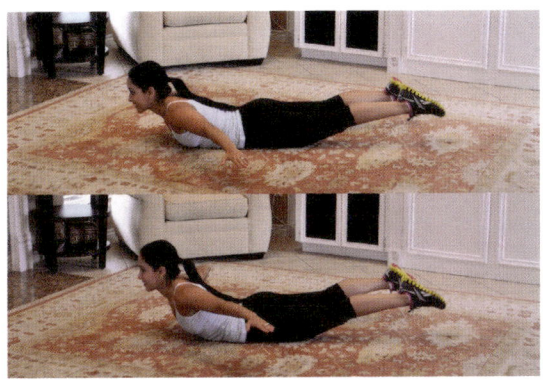

- **DOUBLE PULSE BACK EXTENSION:** Starting position; lie on stomach and extend arms to your side. Ending position; lift chest and shoulders off floor and double pulse on top and release.

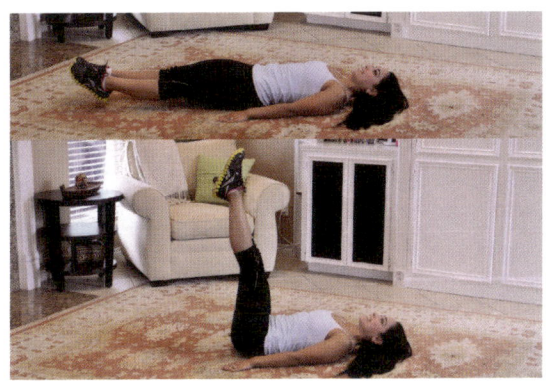

- **DOUBLE LEG LIFTS:** Starting position; lie flat on back with arms to side and legs extended on floor. Ending position; lift legs and point feet to ceiling and release.

- **CARDIO:** Mountain climbers (30-45 seconds)

Circuit 2 (Lower Body)

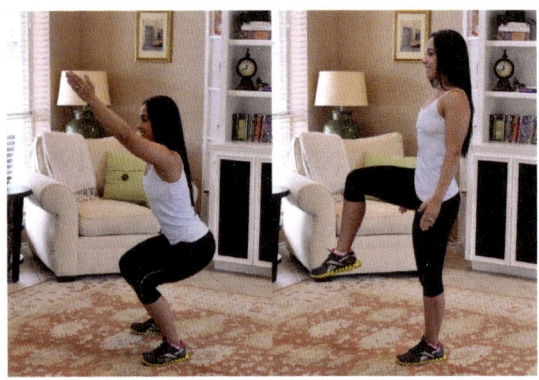

- STANDING LEG LIFTS : Starting position; feet hip width apart with hands on waist. Extend one leg to the back 45-degree angle with foot flexed. Ending position; hold and squeeze glutes and release.

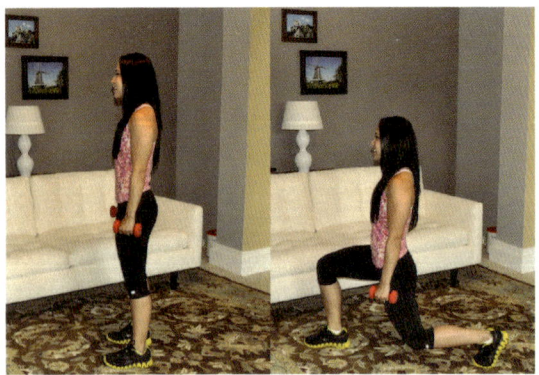

- WALKING LUNGE WITH ALTERNATING LEG EXTENSION: Starting position; one dumbbell in each hand and stand upright. Step forward with one foot. The toes of both feet should be facing straight ahead. Be sure your legs are aligned - your front knee should be aligned with the foot. Ending position; lower your back knee towards the floor. Push back up to the starting position and squeeze glutes then switch. As you switch extend your back leg and left foot off floor.

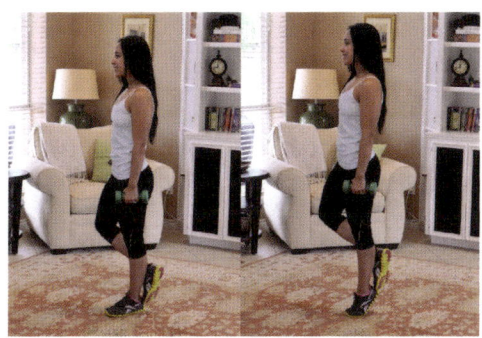

- SINGLE LEG CALF RAISES WITH DUMBBELLS : Starting position; feet hip width apart with toes slightly turned out. Take one foot to opposite ankle. Ending position; lift heel of the foot that's on the floor and release.

- CARDIO: Burpees (10-15 reps): Sit into a squat; kick your feet behind you so you're in a push-up position; pull your feet back in so you're in squat position; stand back up. There are many variations of the burpee to challenge you in different ways (a. when you are in a push-up position, do a push-up before pulling your feet back in b. when you stand back up, jump up instead c. when you jump up, tuck your legs as you jump)

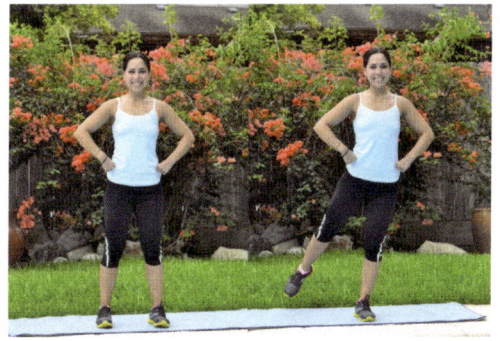

- SINGLE LEG HALF CIRCLE IN HORSE STANCE : Starting position; knees on floor. Lower chest to floor as if you're going into a pushup position (hands shoulder width apart). Bring knees to a 90-degree angle. Ending position; extend one leg to back squeeze glute then release.

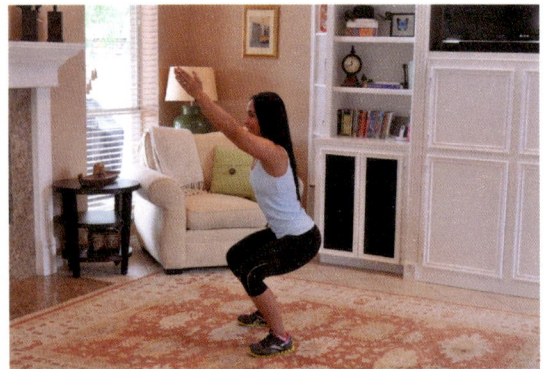

- SQUAT HOLDS: Starting position; bend your knees as if you are sitting into a chair (make sure your knees are over your toes, you should stick your glutes back). Hold the squat for 30 seconds to 1 minute.

- HOVER WITH FOOT LIFT: Starting position; elbows under shoulders with feet hip width apart and push up to your forearms. Ending position; lift one foot slightly and hold then alternate (foot should be at hip level).

- CARDIO: Burpees (10-15 reps)

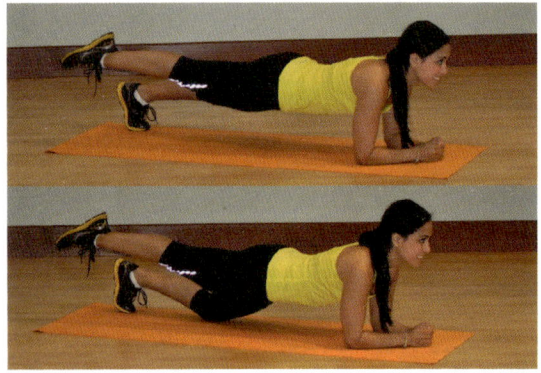

APPENDIX

A. Keeping Track Keeps Me on Track

Week of _____

GEMS FOR THE WEEK		
GEMS	**Plan for Obstacles**	**Successful?**
1.		
2.		
3.		

Food Journal

	Breakfast	Lunch	Dinner	Snacks
Monday				
Time				
Food, Drink, Amount				
Important Note				
Tuesday				
Time				
Food, Drink, Amount				
Important Note				
Wednesday				
Time				
Food, Drink, Amount				
Important Note				
Thursday				
Time				
Food, Drink, Amount				
Important Note				

APPENDIX

Friday				
Time				
Food, Drink, Amount				
Important Note				
Saturday				
Time				
Food, Drink, Amount				
Important Note				
Sunday				
Time				
Food, Drink, Amount				
Important Note				

Physical Activity (What and How Long)

Monday	Tuesday	Wednesday	Thursday	Friday	Saturday	Sunday

Menu Planning for the Week

	Monday	Tuesday	Wednesday	Thursday	Friday	Saturday	Sunday
Breakfast Whole grain, Lean protein or dairy, Fruit							
Lunch Lean protein, Whole grain Veg/Fruit							
Dinner Lean protein Whole grain Veg/Fruit							

B. BMI Chart

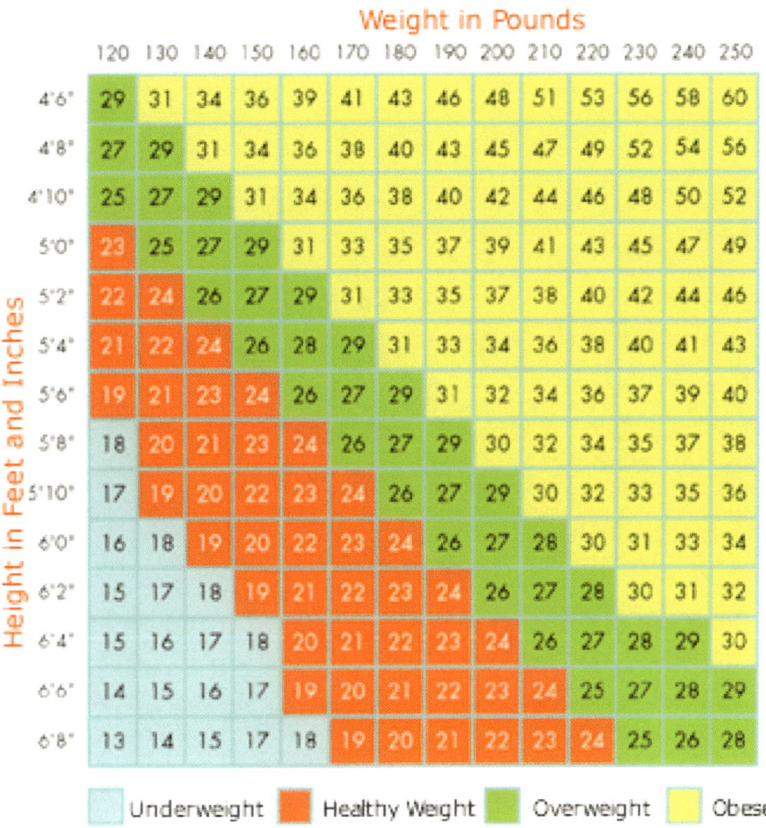

Chart is taken from the Surgeon Generals' website http://www.surgeongeneral.gov/library/calls/obesity/fact_advice.html

Image from http://www.eclevelandclinic.org/bmiPrepare

C. Websites, Apps and Other Great Resources

Here is a compilation of great resources to help you on your journey to a healthier you. These websites, apps and other resources are independent of the South Texas Slim Down, but nonetheless, full of great information.

Websites

1. Academy of Nutrition and Dietetics — http://www.eatright.org
2. American Heart Association — http://www.heart.org
3. Centers for Disease Control and Prevention — http://www.cdc.gov
4. National Diabetes Education Program — http://www.ndep.nih.gov
5. National Heart, Lung, and Blood Institute — http://www.nhlbi.nih.gov
6. US Department of Agriculture — http://www.mypyramid.gov
7. WIN Weight Control Information Network — http://www.win.niddk.nih.gov

Apps

1. MyFitnessPal
2. Fooducate
3. Shopping List (Grocery List) by hensoft
4. Meal Planning and Grocery List by Food on the Table
5. Calorie Tracker by Livestrong
6. Daily Burn Tracker
7. Diet and Food Tracker by Sparkpeople
8. Fast Food Calorie Tracker by Concrete Software, Inc.
9. lolo workout apps

Other Great Resources

1. Weight Watchers
2. Mayo Clinic Diet Book

D.

How to Read Nutrition Labels

1. Serving size-Is the amount stated the amount you are going to eat? If not you may have to double the numbers given.

2. Calories are important! Is it a side item or is it the main entrée? If you plan for a meal 400-500 calories total then you can better judge how and if that is a good choice.

3. Choose items with less saturated fat and as low as possible of trans fat and include more unsaturated fats.

4. Sodium-is it a side item or main entrée? What else will you be eating with it? Aim for no more than 500-700 mg of sodium per meal.

5. Fiber and sugar are carbohydrates. Generally the more fiber the better and less sugar the better. Aim for at least 3 grams of fiber per serving. The total sugar will be listed including natural sugars like the lactose in dairy and the fructose in fruit. There are 4 grams of sugar in one teaspoon.

6. The ingredient list is helpful to find in descending order the most abundant ingredients. So if sugar is one of the first three ingredients or if different forms of sugar are listed throughout, you can be sure that it is providing too much sugar. Refer to list to identify names of sugar.

- Agave nectar, brown sugar, cane sugar, corn sweetener, corn syrup, crystalline fructose, dextrose, fructose, glucose, high-fructose corn syrup, honey, invert sugar, maltose, malt syrup, molasses, raw sugar, sucrose

Healthy Pre-packed Snack Ideas

- low-fat string cheese and a serving of fruit

- handful of nuts and a serving of fruit

- vegetables and hummus

- sliced apple and 2 tbsp peanut butter or almond butter

- yogurt and a serving of fruit

- cottage cheese and a serving of fruit

ENDNOTES

1. Malnick, SD. "The Medical Complications of Obesity." Quart J Med 99 (2006): 565-579
2. Tuomilehto, HP., et al. "Lifestyle Intervention with Weight Reduction: First-line Treatment in Mild Obstructive Sleep Apnea." Am J Respir Crit Care Med 179 (2009): 320-327
3. Purslow, LR., et al. "Energy Intake at Breakfast and Weight Change: Prospective Study of 6,764 Middle-Aged Men and Women." Am J Epid 167 (2008): 167-188
4. Jacobson, BC., et al. "Body-Mass Index and Symptoms of Gastroesophageal Reflux in Women." N Engl J Med 354 (2006): 2340-2348
5. Slavin, JL. "Position of the American Dietetic Association." J Am Diet Assoc 108 (2008): 1716
6. Wood, PD., et al. "Changes in Plasma Lipids and Lipoprotein in Overweight Men during Weight Loss through Dieting as Compared with Exercise." N Engl J Med 319 (1988): 1173-1179
7. Lally, P., Chipperfield, A., and Wardle, J. "Healthy Habits: Efficacy of Simple Advice on Weight Control Based on a Habit-formation Model." Inter J Obes 32 (2008): 700-707
8. In US, 62% Exceed Ideal Weight, 19% at Their Goal Washington, DC (2010) www.gallup.com/poll/144941/exceed-ideal-weight-goal.aspx?version=print
9. Reyes, NR. "Similarities and Differenced Between Weight Loss Maintainers and Regainers: A Qualitative Analysis." J Acad Nutr Diet 112 (2012): 499-505
10. Pham, LB, Taylor, SE. "From Thought to Action: Effects of Process-Versus Outcome-Based Mental Simulations on Performance." Pers Soc Psychol Bull 25 (1999): 250-260
11. US Department of Agriculture, US Department of Health and Human Services. "Dietary Guidelines for Americans 2010." www.health.gov/dietaryguidelines/2010
12. Barr, SB., Wright, JC. "Postprandial Energy Expenditure in Whole-Food and Processed –Food Meals: Implications for Daily Energy Expenditure." Food Nutr Res 54 (2010): 5144

13. Chandalia, M., et al. "Beneficial Effects of High Dietary Fiber Intake in Patients with Type 2 Diabetes Mellitus." New Eng J Med 342 (2000): 1392-1398
14. Brown, L., et al. "Cholesterol-lowering Effects of Dietary Fiber: A Meta-Analysis." Am J Clin Nutr 69 (1999): 30-42
15. Slavin, JL. "Dietary Fiber and Body Weight." Nutr 21 (2005):411-418
16. "Howarth, NC., et al. "Dietary Fiber and Fat are Associated with Excess Weight in Young and Middle Aged US Adults." J Am Diet Assoc 105 (2005): 1365-1372
17. Murphy, M., et al. "Phytonutrient Intake by Adults in the United States in Relation to Fruit and Vegetable Consumption." J Acad Nutr Diet 112 (2012): 222-229
18. Padden-Jones, D., et al. "Protein Weight Management and Satiety." Am J Clin Nutr 87 (2008): 1558s-1561s
19. Willet, WC. "Dietary Fats and Coronary Heart Disease." J Intern Med 42 (2012): 13-14
20. Hu, FB., Manson, JE., Willett, WC. "Types of Dietary Fat and Risk of Coronary Heart Disease: A Critical Review." J Am Coll Nutr 20 (2001): 5-19
21. Whelton, PK., et al. "Effects of Oral Potassium on Blood Pressure: Meta-Analysis of Randomized Controlled Clinical Trials." JAMA 277 (1997): 1624-1632
22. Ross, AC., et al. "The 2011 Dietary Reference Intakes for Calcium and Vitamin D: What Dietetics Practitioners Need to Know." J Am Diet Assoc 111 (2011): 524-527
23. Kavey, RW. "How Sweet It Is: Sugar Sweetened Beverage Consumption, Obesity, and Cardiovascular Risk in Childhood." J Am Diet Assoc 110 (2010):1456-1460
24. Storey, ML., Forshee, RA., Anderson, PA. "Beverage Consumption in the US Population." J Am Diet Assoc 106 (2006):1992-2000
25. Cho, S., et al. "The Effect of Breakfast Type on Total Daily Energy Intake and Body Mass Index: Results from the Third National Health and Nutrition Examination Survey (NHANESIII)." J Am Coll Nutr 22(2003): 296-302
26. Kong, A., et al. "Self-Monitoring and Eating-Related Behaviors are Associated with 12-Month Weight Loss in Postmenopausal Overweight-to Obese Women." J Acad Nutr Diet 112(2012): 1428-1435

Made in the USA
San Bernardino, CA
30 March 2014